**A Hands-On Guide for Local Programs**

# AIDS
## and Your Religious Community

Warren J. Blumenfeld, writer
The Rev. Scott W. Alexander, project director

A Joint Project of the
Unitarian Universalist Association and the
AIDS National Interfaith Network

Production Editor: Katherine Wolff
Copy Editor: Dee Ready
Editorial Assistant: Stephen L'Heureux
Text Designer: Suzanne Morgan
Cover Designer: Bruce Jones

ISBN 1-55896-243-3
Printed in the USA.

10 9 8 7 6 5 4 3 2 1
99 98 97 96 95 94 93 92 91

Library of Congress Cataloging-in-Publication Data
Blumenfeld, Warren J., 1947-

   AIDS and your religious community: a hands-on guide for local programs /
Warren J. Blumenfeld, writer; Scott W. Alexander, project director.
   p.   cm.
   Includes bibliographical references.
   ISBN 1-55896-243-3
   1. AIDS (Disease)—Patients—Pastoral counseling of.
I. Alexander, Scott W.  II. Unitarian Universalist Association.
III. AIDS National Interfaith Network.  IV. Title.
BV4460.7.B58   1991
259'.4—dc20                                          91-28676
                                                     CIP

## Acknowledgments

The Unitarian Universalist Association and the AIDS National Interfaith
Network would like to thank Mr. Albert Goldsmith of Pittsburgh, Pennsylvania, whose generous contribution made this book possible.

We are grateful for the use of material from the following sources:  Earl E.
Shelp and Ronald H. Sunderland, *AIDS and the Church*, The Westminster
Press, Philadelphia, 1987.  Randy Shilts, *And the Band Played On: Politics,
People, and the AIDS Epidemic*, St. Martin's Press, New York, 1987.  C. Everett
Koop in "Do the Right Thing," by Adelman, *Washingtonian*, April, 1990.
National Commission on AIDS, "Panel Says Government Is Not Leading
AIDS Fight," *New York Times*, April 25, 1990.  American Psychiatric Association, *Position Statement Opposing Mandatory Name-Reporting of HIV-Seropositive
Individuals*, November, 1989.  *Boston Globe*, "Report Urges 25% Raise in AIDS
Funding," taken from *Los Angeles Times* wire, March 8, 1991.  Derrick Z.
Jackson, "Courage and Condoms," editorial *Boston Globe*, March 11, 1991.
Derrick Z. Jackson, "Fight AIDS, Not Needles," editorial *Boston Globe*, June 9,
1989.  *The Jersey Journal and Jersey Observer*, "God's Love: A Very Special
Delivery," by Jane Greenstein, August 21, 1989.

# Contents

# Introduction

"AIDS is a human disease that can and does afflict all groups of people in our society. Illness and disease are not limited to certain people or certain groups of people. We have been given an opportunity to show God's love manifested in us, as we minister to those with AIDS. . . . All of us are made in the image of God. How we reach out to [persons with AIDS] also reflects how we reach out to God. We can no longer say that the disease does not affect me or my family or neighbor. We are all related."
—The Union of Black Episcopalians' AIDS Task Force

On December 4, 1989, many of our foremost religious leaders gathered at the Carter Presidential Center in Atlanta for a national symposium called "AIDS: The Moral Imperative." More than 100 leaders from some twenty religious traditions met in an atmosphere of urgency and resolve.

The assembled participants listened while experts described the AIDS crisis and religious leaders articulated the scriptural message to care for those members of the human family who are ill and in need of comfort and support. These same participants drafted and ratified *The Atlanta Declaration*. According to this document, today's religious communities must do the following:

- "Embody and proclaim hope, life, and healing in the midst of suffering."
- "Assure that all whose lives are affected" by AIDS "will have access to compassion, nonjudgmental care, respect, support, and assistance."
- "Generate a prophetic vision of society in which the 'general welfare' becomes the abiding obligation of public, private, and voluntary sectors of society."
- "Provide accurate and comprehensive information for the public regarding HIV transmission, related behavior patterns, and means of prevention."
- "Transform public attitudes and policies so that adequate care and appropriate preventative measures will be available for all people in need."

*The Atlanta Declaration* calls for "creative action" among all religious institutions as they accept the responsibilities listed in the document.

In response to *The Atlanta Declaration*, the AIDS Action and Information Program of the Unitarian Universalist Association and the AIDS National Interfaith Network (with the generous assistance of members of many religious communities throughout the United States and Canada), have produced this book. As a hands-on manual, it provides step-by-step practical guidance and information that will help your faith community initiate or expand an AIDS/HIV ministry.

As you know, faith communities across the continent have mobilized their resources to create hundreds of programs through which members minister to those affected by AIDS. Section 1 of this working manual offers you a sampling of these creative ministry programs. You can duplicate these models or modify them to meet the needs of your local community. Both diverse and intriguing, the models offer everything from pastoral to personal support, day-care to dental services, housing to hospice care, food shopping to "meals on wheels," bookkeeping to housekeeping aid, legal to medical assistance. All the programs featured in this manual are fully identified at the back (see Services and Organizations in Section 4, the Resources section). These listings (both alphabetical and by state) include program addresses, phone numbers, and—whenever possible—the name of a contact person, so that you can get additional information.

The pastoral models described here rest on the universal religious and moral imperative to feed the hungry, give drink to the thirsty, welcome the stranger, clothe the naked, care for the sick, and visit the imprisoned (Matthew 25:31-46). Through their varied ministries, the faith communities represented by these models help children, women, and men empower themselves. People living with AIDS need to recognize and use the resources of their local communities, develop their own personal resources, control their own decisions, solve their own problems, and achieve their own goals. And those who assist people living with AIDS face the difficult challenge of allowing those people to be as independent as possible.

Section 2 of this manual provides information on fundamental issues you must address before undertaking AIDS ministry—as well as many practical suggestions for how to begin your chosen response to AIDS. This section helps you to do the following:

- consider the requirements of AIDS ministry;
- assess the needs of persons living with AIDS/HIV in your local community;
- evaluate your group's financial, material, and human resources;
- focus your resources on one manageable project;
- recruit and support volunteers;
- train and educate volunteers.

Section 3, which outlines some AIDS-related issues and highlights a number of social justice strategies, helps you consider public-policy issues related to AIDS/HIV on local, state, and federal levels. It includes a variety of options, some more controversial than others.

Finally, Section 4 offers resource information that will help you educate your faith community about AIDS/HIV.

Because each faith community or interfaith coalition is at a different stage in its AIDS ministry, this manual will open new and uncharted territory for you or will help you to assess the program you already have in place. The basic philosophy behind this book is that you can best accomplish ministry when you proceed in a thoughtful, step-by-step sequence without short cuts. Whatever your position in the process of AIDS ministry, you'll want to carefully review and consider each section of this manual before proceeding further with your outreach to those living with AIDS and with the diagnosis of HIV+.

# ONE

# The Models

Individual faith communities or interfaith coalitions can consider many different kinds of AIDS-related programs. Your project can focus solely on AIDS, you can incorporate an AIDS component within an existing project (like housing for the needy), or you can institute a new project with a multifocused agenda that includes AIDS.

The following pages present models of existing programs—including personal support, food and meals, housing and hospices, and drop-in and day-care centers. The quotations and suggestions that accompany the main text apply to the program models in which they appear. (To preserve the privacy of those involved, we do not always identify the speaker.) Also, all working models are fully identified starting on page 104.

Within the personal support section, you will find models that offer pastoral counseling, support therapy groups, "buddy" programs, worship services of hope and healing, and a "Names Quilt" project.

Within the food projects, you will find food pantries (also called "food banks") that involve coordinating the collection of nonperishable food and establishing mechanisms for distribution; food kitchens ("meals on wheels") that involve the gathering, preparation, and distribution of food; and monthly/weekly dinners offered at a religious building or other site (a hospital AIDS unit or a hospice, for example).

Within the housing and hospice models, you will find AIDS houses purchased by a group for independent living and moderate care facilities; AIDS houses for rent or lease to provide independent living and moderate care facilities; hospices that provide skilled nursing care; and home care that provides support for daily living from nursing to visitation.

Within the drop-in and day-care section, you will find day care for HIV+ adults as well as day care for HIV+ children (or children of HIV-infected parents).

As you read through these models, you'll note many other kinds of additional support: transportation (to and from doctor's appointments, for example), cooking, shopping, walking pets, massage, cutting hair, low-cost medical care, low-cost dental care, banking and other financial services, legal services, advocacy through the social service bureaucracy, and foster and adoptive parenting to HIV+ infants and children. In addition you'll discover methods of raising funds such as an "AIDS Walk" to raise money for a local AIDS organization, cultural or fine art performances, and direct-mail solicitations.

# Personal Support

"Where there is great love there are always miracles."
—Willa Cather

## CHRISTIAN MINISTERIAL ALLIANCE, INC. • Little Rock, AR

The Christian Ministerial Alliance, Inc., is an ecumenical religious fellowship consisting of clergy representatives from nine denominations: Church of God in Christ, African Methodist Episcopal, African Methodist Episcopal Zion, Christian Methodist Episcopal, United Methodist Church, Church of Christ Holiness USA, Presbyterian USA, Baptist, and Muslim.

The Alliance operates on two fronts. First, it makes emergency referrals for persons who need food, shelter, clothing, health care, and psychological counseling. Second, it educates the public on important issues such as AIDS, housing availability, racism, sexism, and other vital topics that affect the quality of life of persons living in Pulaski County, Arkansas.

### Background and Development

The Christian Ministerial Alliance, Inc., was founded in 1977 to educate its congregations about issues of concern to people in the state of Arkansas. The AIDS Education/Prevention component began in June of 1989 because Alliance members were concerned about the disproportionate number of AIDS cases in communities of color. Members of the Alliance recognized an opportunity to utilize the influence of the church to combat this problem.

Through the Arkansas State Health Department, the Alliance obtained a grant from the Centers for Disease Control in Atlanta to cover start-up expenses. Eventually, the Alliance hired a part-time employee to oversee volunteers from local churches and health-care professionals to facilitate a series of AIDS education/prevention workshops.

### Organization, Operation, and Resources

The AIDS Education/Prevention Project of the Christian Ministerial Alliance, Inc., coordinates AIDS education workshops at member churches throughout Pulaski County and central Arkansas. These workshops last from three to five hours. The format of each workshop consists of a medical presentation (usually by a health professional or other trained staff person) followed by a question-and-answer session. Sometimes the presenter assigns a role-playing activity or other form of exercise and, on occasion, shows a film. A minister from the Alliance facilitates a theological dialogue on the topic of AIDS

*"We got a call a couple of months ago from a young lady whose brother died of AIDS. Her family didn't have any money to take care of the funeral expenses and they couldn't find an undertaker to take care of the body because of fear. Through our network we found an undertaker who would do it. We then went to our congregations, who took care of the expenses. The response from that family made all of our efforts worthwhile. We've become thankful for small victories like this one."*

Rev. Don Gibson
St. Peter's Rock Baptist Church
Little Rock, AR

> *"By working with this AIDS project, I can plainly see that a change in the way the religious community thinks has taken place. Yes, there are still far too many who say that this disease is God's punishment for sin. However, unlike when we started, more people are asking and trying to find out what they can do to stop the spread of AIDS as well as help the folks with AIDS and their families. I think that this is what Jesus wants us to do."*

(using compassion versus taking a judgmental stance, for example) and offers biblical insights meant to shatter any lingering thoughts that AIDS is a form of divine retribution. The presenter distributes materials (pamphlets, posters, booklets) to raise the awareness of participants. As a follow-up to the workshop, the Alliance assists local churches in developing their own AIDS education component.

The Alliance also sponsors peer counseling. Alliance members train volunteers to go into local communities, predominantly in the inner city, where the incidence of HIV infection is growing, and offer information and counseling to women of color of childbearing age who are at risk for HIV.

The Alliance also makes referrals and offers direct assistance for people with AIDS and their families in times of emergency. According to Rev. Gibson: "We are sometimes asked to give financial assistance. We go into our pockets; we go to our congregations to help people pay rent, to pay for medicine, to help take care of funeral expenses. We also offer emotional support and counseling. We make referrals; we talk to the family and sometimes to the person's minister when we are requested to do so. We help widen the person's support system."

The Alliance has collaborated with other local groups, such as Community Organization for Poverty Elimination, Black Community Developers, Regional AIDS Interfaith Network, and the United States Conference of Black Mayors.

Volunteers are members and officers of local church groups (called auxiliaries), such as The Brotherhood, Missionary Society, Willing Worker's Club, Deacon Board—plus local ministers. The workshop participants are concerned parishioners as well as local health professionals from such groups as the Visiting Nurses Association and the Black Nurses Association.

Financial support has come from the Center for Disease Control in Atlanta, and from denominational agencies, private foundation, local businesses, fund-raising benefits, and other projects. Local businesses and churches donate equipment and space.

## EPISCOPAL CARING RESPONSE TO AIDS, INC. • Washington, DC

The Episcopal Caring Response to AIDS (ECRA) is a nonprofit coalition operated by representatives from thirty-two Episcopal parishes and related organizations in the Washington, DC, area. This organization provides support to those affected by AIDS/HIV regardless of religious affiliation. ECRA offers programs that include a home and a food bank for persons with AIDS, pediatric respite care, an AIDS chaplaincy, parish education, and spiritual retreats.

## Background and Development

In Anaheim, California, in 1985, delegates to the annual Episcopal Church Convention passed a resolution calling on the church to support the efforts of the gay, lesbian, and bisexual communities in working to end the spread of AIDS. Following this resolution, a handful of churches in the Washington, DC, area organized the Episcopal Caring Response to AIDS, Inc., in June 1986. After contacting the Whitman-Walker Clinic—the area's leading AIDS service organization—to assess local needs, the members of ECRA decided to assist in the funding of a home for persons with AIDS.

## Organization, Operation, and Resources

An all-volunteer board of directors, which is composed of two members from each Episcopal parish and from each organization belonging to ECRA, governs the coalition. A full-time administrator coordinates the day-to-day activities. Other staff members include an administrative secretary and executive director. The program is funded through individual contributions.

ECRA sponsors a broad range of activities. For example, it provides funding for the Michael Haass House for persons with AIDS. Named for a local Episcopal organist who died of an AIDS-related illness, the Michael Haass House was opened in the District of Columbia in September 1986. It is home to people who are well enough to live independently but who cannot support themselves financially because of their illness. Parishioners furnish the home with donated items and help supply food and clothing to its residents. The Whitman-Walker Clinic manages the home.

The pediatric respite-care program recruits and trains volunteers to assist and support the families of HIV-infected children. Volunteers baby-sit, run errands, do household chores, and lend a sympathetic ear. The volunteers work both in the children's homes and in a respite-care center in downtown Washington.

ECRA employs Rev. Jerry Anderson, an Episcopal priest in the Diocese of Washington, to offer spiritual guidance and support to persons with AIDS/HIV and their loved ones. Rev. Anderson, who extends support regardless of a person's religious affiliation, makes home and hospital visits, offers counseling, leads a spiritual support group and healing services, plans and officiates at funerals, and provides other services to persons with AIDS.

ECRA is also involved in the area of AIDS education. Through speakers, panelists, films, discussions, and printed material, ECRA helps parishes and other groups answer questions about AIDS. The coalition offers educational training to clergy, staff, and lay persons in the Diocese of Washington. Using respected theological, pastoral, and medical authorities, ECRA's educational seminars address a variety of concerns. The presenters tailor the content, length, and format of a seminar to the interests and concerns of each parish.

> Ask all members of the support group to commit to long-term, active involvement. Stability, trust, continuity, and community are important concerns to persons with AIDS, many of whom have experienced a profound sense of loss.

*"As a year of searching came to an end, I realized that what I was looking for I always had—myself. When I finally accepted that self, all the defenses, the fears, the tensions vanished. The three retreats I attended made such a gradual discovery possible. How else would I have learned about unconditional love?"*

ECRA also maintains an AIDS resource library open to churches and other religious bodies.

ECRA works closely with the Whitman-Walker Clinic Food Bank, which provides basic food items at no cost to people living with AIDS. Volunteers pick up and deliver donated food.

ECRA and Damien Ministries, a Roman Catholic AIDS service organization based in Washington, DC, jointly sponsor spiritual retreats for people with AIDS/HIV infection. The two organizations hold retreats at a pastoral center in West Virginia and in Maryland. Forty to fifty people gather for four days to explore issues such as finding spiritual strength in the face of life-threatening illness; coping with loss, guilt, stigma, and anger; overcoming isolation; experiencing intimacy; and seeking a loving creator despite experiences of alienation from religious institutions. These retreats inspire and empower spiritual growth for people living with AIDS/HIV in a context of community building and unconditional love.

Men and women, gay and straight, of varied races, diverse educational and economic status, and spiritual backgrounds participate in these retreats. Some participants come with loved ones, buddies, or family members. Some are in recovery from addiction. All have found themselves in spiritual crisis as a result of their diagnosis.

The retreats draw upon traditional and innovative methods and embrace diverse spiritual heritages. Activities include thematic presentations, creative exercises, worship, relaxation, play, and group discussion. Twelve-step recovery groups are also available. Participants, who meet in the full group, in small groups, or in one-to-one interaction, experience varied types of formats—from peer support and group discussion to drawing, dance, and music.

A resource team of lay and ordained persons from ECRA, Damien, and the larger AIDS service community, including persons with HIV infection, lead the retreats. Depending on the specific activities planned, individuals from local, regional, and national organizations offer their expertise.

In addition to these programs, ECRA volunteers undertake occasional short-term activities, such as collecting Christmas gifts and cooking holiday dinners for people with AIDS. ECRA has also provided speakers and additional resources in support of the Presiding Bishop's annual AIDS Day of Prayer.

## LAZARUS PROJECT • Hollywood, CA

The Lazarus Project of the West Hollywood Presbyterian Church coordinates a Christian AIDS support group for people with AIDS/HIV and assists other churches in conducting AIDS education and in forming similar groups.

## Background and Development

As the AIDS crisis grew in Los Angeles, a number of community organizations emerged to offer assistance and support for persons with AIDS/HIV, their families, and their loved ones. Soon, however, these organizations discovered that no one offered support for Christian persons with AIDS/HIV and that most mainstream Christian churches were visibly absent in providing pastoral care to persons with AIDS/HIV and their loved ones.

The Lazarus Project of the West Hollywood Presbyterian Church eventually coordinated a support group that would answer that need. Founded in 1977 (before the AIDS epidemic was even identified), the Lazarus Project welcomes members of the gay, lesbian, and bisexual communities and serves as a ministry of reconciliation. Just as Jesus called Lazarus from his tomb—over objections—so, too, the Lazarus Project calls lesbians, gay males, and bisexual people from their closets despite longstanding objections from church and society.

Persons with AIDS organized the spiritual support group of the Lazarus Project themselves. Church members believed that if those most affected by AIDS developed a support group, their commitment to it would be stronger than if a mandate were handed down to them by people who thought they needed support. The working philosophy of this group is that persons living with AIDS must control their own support and their own spirituality.

## Organization, Operation, and Resources

Two members of the church—one clergy person and one lay person—facilitate the spiritual support group for persons with AIDS/HIV. The group meets for prayer, Bible study, retreats, and the celebration of Communion. Members come from diverse backgrounds and life-styles. The group meets every other week in the homes of the participants. This personalizes the experience, gives the members an opportunity to meet in different environments, and provides safety. Members decide the boundaries to set for inclusion of new members, such as persons with a full diagnosis of AIDS, persons with AIDS-Related Complex (ARC), persons with HIV infection, spouses, support givers, families and/or parents, and so on.

Through contact with local AIDS projects and by referral of care providers, the church and other churches and denominations in the area learn about the group. One facilitator serves as the contact person and meets with interested parties prior to their joining the group.

Through a grant from Presbyterian Women, the Lazarus Project has sponsored the production of an educational film geared to congregations and universities. The film, *Pastoral Care for Persons with AIDS,* documents the story of West Hollywood Presbyterian Church's involvement with AIDS. With the film comes a study guide which answers some common questions related to AIDS. The film and study guide are available upon request.

**If your group decides to be open to *any* HIV+ individual, expect the presence of "difficult" members. A facilitator needs to assert her/himself and protect the group from abusive behavior.**

The problem of group depression is naturally exacerbated when a member dies. If this happens, be sure to provide time for sharing both grief and anxiety. When members report on their week, encourage them to end on a positive note by sharing something they feel good about. If you are the facilitator, be alert to the mood of the group and be prepared to use process skills to deal with group depression.

Other Lazarus projects include the following: ongoing Bible study and worship at the church; counseling for lesbian, bisexual, and gay parishioners and their families and friends; worship services at the Los Angeles County jail for gay inmates who are prevented from attending services with other inmates; coordination of educational conferences on lesbian, bisexual, and gay concerns; coordination of award dinners honoring Californians for outstanding work in promoting gay/lesbian/bisexual spirituality or reconciliation with predominantly heterosexual communities; and publication of *Lazarus Rising*, a quarterly newsletter that chronicles the work of the project.

## SOLIDARITY • Schenectady, NY

This program provides peer support for people in the Schenectady/Albany area who are HIV+ or have ARC or AIDS.

### Background and Development

Around 1987 many people in this community realized that AIDS was a growing problem. The local council of churches, area school boards, a newly formed AIDS task force, and other agencies mobilized to conduct education and prevention programs. This group produced AIDS prevention posters and television spots and scheduled talks on AIDS.

Neither the churches nor the community agencies, however, were interested in providing services or programs for people who were HIV+ or for persons living with AIDS. Moreover, by stressing the dangers of HIV infection through its focus on education, the work of these organizations had the unintended effect of causing the general public to fear those already infected. This, plus the scare tactics used by the media in reporting AIDS, resulted in acts of discrimination against HIV-infected individuals. For example, landlords evicted some people from their apartments once their HIV status became known and area dentists denied dental care to others.

Aware that an HIV support group was desperately needed, the Social Responsibility Committee of the Unitarian Society of Schenectady sponsored such a group, gave it a name, and budgeted $400. The committee decided that Rev. Charles Slap would facilitate the group, which would meet weekly in the evening for two hours at the church parsonage and that the group would be limited to people who tested HIV+.

Next, the committee needed to find a way to inform the HIV+ population about the group without incurring negative attention. To protect participant anonymity and avoid harassment, group coordinators decided not to make public the meeting times and the locations. The coordinators sent notices to the AIDS units of area hospitals, physicians who treated HIV, the Gay

Community Center, community health centers, and selected community agencies. The notice announced the formation of an HIV support group sponsored by the church, and gave the phone number of the church (with contact names).

## Organization, Operation, and Resources

The membership of this peer support group includes heterosexuals, gay males, bisexuals, lesbians, African Americans, Latino/as, Caucasians, women and men, people who are healthy, and people who are sick. When an individual calls to seek information about the group, the minister or contact person asks the caller who referred them, their HIV status, and their first name. If the caller reports that she or he is HIV+, the contact person invites the caller to the next support meeting.

The core support group now consists of about 20 individuals with an average weekly attendance of 12. Over 100 individuals have participated in the group since its founding and many nonregulars come back occasionally.

Members provide their own transportation to and from meetings. After attending a meeting or two, almost everyone arranges to be part of a carpool. If an individual does not have transportation, the group encourages him or her to take a taxi to the meeting. The facilitator either pays the cab driver or reimburses the member.

The group subscribes to *Body Positive*, a journal geared to the needs of HIV+ people. In addition, other publications, such as *The AIDS Treatment News*, are available at no charge. The group spends about $400 per year, mostly for literature and transportation. This money comes from the social-action budget of the church. An AIDS-related foundation donates $100.

At the meetings, members, in turn, are given the opportunity to report on their week by sharing details about their emotional and physical health and other significant aspects of their lives. For the last half hour of the meeting, the members discuss a topic they selected at the beginning of the session. On occasion, the group suspends the usual format to provide time for an outside speaker or a film. Refreshments are served at the close of the session.

Because everyone in the group is HIV+ and the group admits no one who is HIV-negative, members share and bond to an extent that would be impossible with an "outsider" present. Speakers—such as medical specialists or persons with AIDS doing well on an alternate treatment—are invited only with the consensus of the group.

An official of a local AIDS council suggested that this support group might want to separate those who are sick from those who are healthy. The group members strongly resented this suggestion. They feel a strong sense of loyalty to each other and are unwilling to abandon an individual because of illness. In fact, when someone is hospitalized, the members ensure that he or she receives visits.

**Remember that facilitators and support group members should maintain absolute confidentiality concerning the makeup of the group, the names of the participants, and the details of their group sharing.**

In conjunction with an AIDS activist group in a nearby city, group members take part in monthly social outings, ranging from pool parties to bowling and barbecues. Because several members are in recovery from drug dependency, the group prohibits alcohol at its meetings and at social functions.

Some members report that this support group is the most loving, caring community they have ever experienced. Within this group they feel safe, can speak freely, and share their anxieties and frustrations.

Although subsequent community efforts to form other HIV support groups have met with modest success, this support group continues to demonstrate vitality, enthusiasm, and a strong sense of family. A major contributing factor for this vitality may be that the group is closed to all those who are not HIV+.

## PASTORAL CARE REFERRAL SERVICE • West Newton, MA

The Pastoral Care Referral Service of Interfaith AIDS Ministry links persons with AIDS, persons who are HIV+, their families, and their friends to volunteer pastoral care givers in the greater Boston area. The program also provides emergency supplemental aid and coordinates spiritual retreats.

### Background and Development

Serving as chaplain at Massachusetts General Hospital in Boston, Rev. Katrina Finley realized that the spiritual needs of people with AIDS were unmet once they left the hospital. In 1987 she founded the Interfaith AIDS Ministry (IAM). When a local AIDS organization dropped pastoral care from its services, IAM initiated conversations with agencies, hospital chaplaincies, AIDS organizations, and home health-care providers. The need for referral services was obvious, so IAM founded the Pastoral Care Referral Service.

### Organization, Operation, and Resources

The cooperating AIDS organizations, hospitals, agencies, and hospices refer clients who request pastoral care to IAM. IAM then refers clients to appropriate agencies for pastoral services, thus making available experienced, trained, and professional care givers where and when they are needed. IAM keeps a log of references and service.

Participating volunteers include clergy and laity from Roman Catholic, Anglican, Protestant, and Jewish traditions who are required to have AIDS training and/or experience working with HIV-related issues. The program is based on clusters, that is, a group of congregations in geographical proximity committed to working with home health-care agencies and other AIDS organizations.

IAM functions solely as a referral service and does not engage in any direct counseling or care on its own. Referral services include the following: individual pastoral counseling, family or group pastoral counseling, spiritual guidance (in tradition of choice as requested), chaplaincy to care givers, home visits (in tradition of choice as requested), hospital and hospice visitation as requested (in tradition of choice), sacramental care, support for healing services, religious services as requested, grief counseling, funeral planning, crisis intervention, pastoral training programs, friendly conversation, and presence in AIDS organizations as mutually agreeable.

With the help of volunteers, IAM also provides emergency supplemental aid in the form of food, linen and adult diapers, clothing, personal items, and transportation. IAM members conduct AIDS educational seminars for congregations and plan spiritual retreats for anyone affected by HIV.

All pastoral care providers and delegates from the referring agencies (including representatives from among the clients) are members of the Pastoral Care Program Council, which meets every four months. These business meetings discuss the direction and effectiveness of the program, make recommendations to the IAM Board of Directors, and promote mutual relations between faith traditions and organizations that work with concerns involving AIDS. An executive director manages the program.

The Second Church of West Newton, Massachusetts, provides office space. Funding comes from foundation grants and individual donations specifically earmarked for the operating costs of the Pastoral Care Referral Services and for spiritual retreats.

**If you are establishing a referral service, be sure that you do not engage in direct counseling or care of persons affected by HIV. And do not accept responsibility for the care actually rendered by professionals to persons who are referred. Take every opportunity to convey to secular agencies how valuable religious/spiritual care is to many persons affected by HIV.**

# UNITARIAN UNIVERSALIST
# METRO MINISTRY OF ATLANTA • Atlanta, GA

The Unitarian Universalist Metro Ministry of Atlanta provides pastoral care, counseling, and emotional support for persons with AIDS/HIV, their friends, and their families. In addition, the ministry makes referrals to other agencies and provides memorial services.

## Background and Development

The Unitarian Universalist Congregation of Atlanta recruited Rev. Joe Chancey to serve in the volunteer position of affiliate minister for AIDS action. In this position, he soon realized that the work could easily become full-time if he could find funding. In 1985 he gathered ministers and lay persons from several local Unitarian Universalist congregations and formed the Unitarian

Universalist Metro Ministry of Atlanta. Initial funding came from the Unitarian Universalist Denominational Grants Panel and from contributions and pledges, primarily from local Unitarian Universalist congregations. Rev. Chancey was initially hired at one-third time, then one-half time, and finally full time.

### Organization, Operation, and Resources

The program provides ongoing services tailored to suit the individual needs of the clients. Among these services are short- and long-term counseling, referrals, and occasional transportation to appointments.

The ministry also sponsors weekend spiritual retreats for persons who are HIV+. Members participate in trust exercises, meditation, yoga, and Sunday morning worship services. A "cleansing fire" exercise involves participants tossing an item they brought from home into a fire. This action symbolizes the freeing of their minds by literally letting go of something.

Unfortunately, local funding for this project did not increase as grant money decreased, and the paid position held by Rev. Chancey was eliminated in December 1990. Having to postpone services saddened ministry members. Those who sit on the board of directors hope to resurrect the project in a scaled-down version.

## WINGSPAN MINISTRY • St. Paul, MN

Wingspan is a welcoming Lutheran congregation for gay, lesbian, and bisexual people and their families and friends. It helps those who have experienced neglect or rejection at the hands of other religious organizations "to come home again." The ministry supports, empowers, and nurtures "like the mother eagle who teaches her young to fly"—hence the name Wingspan. Some of the work of this ministry centers on the issue of AIDS.

### Background and Development

In 1977 a referendum was placed before the voters of St. Paul, Minnesota, which sought to exclude gay males, lesbians, and bisexual people from protections covered under that city's human rights ordinance. The pastors and leadership of the St. Paul-Reformation Lutheran Church publicly opposed the passage of this referendum. Nonetheless, the referendum passed.

In March 1982, the Church Council of the congregation voted unanimously to sanction the establishment of Wingspan as a ministry visibly committed to meeting the needs of its own members (gay, lesbian, bisexual, heterosexual) and to lifting up Christian concern for lesbian, bisexual, and gay persons in other congregations and in society as a whole.

## Organization, Operation, and Resources

Wingspan, which works in cooperation with the Lutheran AIDS Ministry and the AIDS Interfaith Council of Minnesota, directs its energies to pastoral care, education and consultation, interpretation, and witness and advocacy.

Pastoral care centers directly on the needs of gay males, lesbians, and bisexual people (some of whom are living with AIDS/HIV) and those whose lives are touched by these individuals. Services include counseling and developing a supportive community. Wingspan conducts "The Service of the Word for Healing," a special AIDS service of prayer in the Lutheran tradition.

Wingspan serves as an informational/educational resource to congregational members, other clergy, and church structures with respect to gay/lesbian/bisexual and AIDS issues, especially as they relate to growth in faith and the community of faith. Wingspan hopes that a growing openness toward gay/lesbian/bisexual persons and their families will develop within other congregations. The organization also interprets the vision and intent of its ministry to the congregation, other congregations, church structures, and to gay/lesbian/bisexual persons, their families, and their friends.

Witness and advocacy efforts within Wingspan include providing support, intervention, and encouragement to the community and to the broader church and society. This is done in the hope of advancing a better quality of life and faith for gay/lesbian/bisexual persons. The ministry also works to develop progressive AIDS public policy. In addition, Wingspan played a major role in bringing the NAMES Project Quilt to Minnesota and produced a film and theater piece focusing on AIDS.

**Hosting a quilting bee can be an excellent entry project for members of your faith community who may be nervous about hands-on AIDS ministry. Quilting bees are easily intergenerational, and often stimulate further AIDS ministry. If your group is interested, contact the NAMES Project Foundation (see the Resources section).**

## THE NAMES PROJECT AIDS MEMORIAL QUILT • San Francisco, CA

Based in San Francisco, the NAMES Project AIDS Memorial Quilt coordinates the production of quilt panels, which, when pieced together, serve as memorials to all those who have died from AIDS-related illnesses.

## Background and Development

The idea of the quilt originated with Cleve Jones in response to a candlelight memorial for Harvey Milk and George Moscone, in November 1985. A year and a half later, in June 1987, Jones teamed up with Mike Smith to organize the NAMES Project Foundation. They began to sponsor the making of quilt panels to memorialize those who had died of the epidemic. As the epidemic continued to rage, word of the quilt spread.

Response was immediate and widespread. People in each of the cities most affected by the epidemic—New York, Los Angeles, and San Francisco—sent quilt panels to the San Francisco workshop in memory of their loved ones. The gay and lesbian community and their friends were especially generous, rapidly filling "wish lists" for sewing machines, office supplies, and volunteers.

On October 11, 1987, the NAMES Project displayed the quilt for the first time. People from all walks of life gathered on the Mall in Washington, DC. There they joined in groups of four to unfold and place on the ground large blocks of brightly colored panels created by friends, lovers, partners, and family members of people who had died of AIDS. Stitched or written on to the panels were souvenirs and images that were significant to those who were memorialized. Together, the quilt covered a space just larger than two football fields and included 1,920 panels. During the ceremony, people read aloud the 1,920 names of men, women, teenagers, children, and infants who had died of AIDS. A half a million people visited the quilt that weekend.

Since its first public display, the quilt has been seen by millions of people around the globe. Every day new panels from all over the world arrive at the NAMES Project workshop in San Francisco, where they are sewn into the quilt by volunteers. Today the quilt includes more than 14,000 panels, weighs 16 tons, and—when displayed together—covers an area the size of almost nine football fields.

## Organization, Operation, and Resources

The NAMES Project continues to display the quilt, across the United States and overseas, to encourage visitors to better understand and respond to the AIDS epidemic, to provide a positive means of expression for those mourning the death of a loved one, and to raise vital community funds for people living with HIV infection, ARC, and AIDS.

Faith communities become involved in the quilt project in a number of ways. Some host a display of quilt panels. Other faith communities or interfaith groups also hold a quilting bee for people who want to create panels for loved ones who have died from AIDS. The Arlington Street Church in Boston (Unitarian Universalist) hosted a weekly quilting bee for several years. On the designated evening, church members and friends would ensure that everything needed for making panels was available: information on the function of panels, many kinds and colors of fabric, sewing machines, and the expertise of people familiar with sewing and quilting. The quilting bee has since moved to the Boston Living Center, a day-care facility for persons affected by AIDS, and continues as a vital and needed weekly event for the people of Boston.

# Food and Meals

"Be not forgetful to entertain strangers: for thereby some have entertained angels unawares."

—Hebrews 13:1-2

## AIDS COMMITTEE • New York, NY

The AIDS Committee at Congregation B'nai Jeshurun in New York City coordinates festive lunches and holiday parties, hospital brunches and volunteer visits, and interfaith activities for people with AIDS/HIV and their loved ones.

### Background and Development

The rabbis and some members of Congregation B'nai Jeshurun synagogue were disappointed at what they perceived to be the slow response by the Jewish community to the AIDS crisis. They found also that many Jewish people with AIDS/HIV, as well as their loved ones, felt ostracized by the Jewish community when they most needed spiritual support. So in 1989, a committee formed to give spiritual comfort to those with AIDS/HIV and their loved ones, regardless of their religious affiliation, and to welcome Jewish people with AIDS/HIV into the congregation.

### Organization, Operation, and Resources

The AIDS Committee at Congregation B'nai Jeshurun synagogue coordinates three interrelated projects. The first consists of festive Shabbat luncheons on Saturday afternoons and spiritual gatherings around Jewish holidays. In total, the committee conducts about ten such events each year for people with AIDS/HIV, their loved ones, and their health-care providers.

In the past, anywhere from 30 to 135 people have attended these special events held in the vestry of the synagogue. Volunteers from the congregation serve the meal. A rabbi leads the gathering in prayer, and local musicians perform. On occasion, members of New York City's Gay Men's Chorus serenade the diners.

Currently Congregation B'nai Jeshurun does not have adequate kitchen facilities to prepare large quantities of food, so they purchase food already prepared. A generous grant provided by the Paul Rappaport Foundation and donations from members of the congregation fund the luncheon. Press releases and direct mailings sent to individuals and some 150 social service agencies in the New York City area publicize the luncheons.

*"What this is all about is needing and caring for one another. You may come here because you have AIDS or are HIV+ and need some comfort from us, but we also need you. When we leave here on Shabbat afternoon, we leave feeling that you have greatly enriched our lives. We leave feeling that all of us have comforted one another as we each face our own tragedies and our own mortality."*

**Rabbi Rolando Matelon**
**Congregation B'nai Jeshurun**
**New York, NY**

**Plan to spend a lot of effort locating the people you want to serve—because they might be hard to reach. Also, extend aid to families, partners, and health-care workers as well as PWAs.**

The AIDS Committee at B'nai Jeshurun also joins with three local churches to serve Sunday brunch to inpatients with AIDS/HIV at St. Luke's Roosevelt Hospital. Each organization coordinates one Sunday of every month in turn. Volunteers prepare the food and serve approximately 70 to 80 people in the hospital lounge and in their rooms. Along with providing the meals on designated Sundays, members of the four congregations lead patients in an interfaith prayer service.

The third project sponsored by the Congregation B'nai Jeshrun involves volunteers visiting hospitals on Saturday afternoon to give support to people with AIDS of all denominations. Most though not all, of the volunteers are congregation members and some are themselves persons with AIDS. Thus, volunteers have the opportunity of practicing the ancient tradition of Bikur Cholim (visiting the sick), which is a biblical commandment. Volunteers sign up for visits on a rotating basis with designated team captains (members of the AIDS Committee who coordinate this project).

After talking with parents of persons with AIDS, committee members have discovered that a support group designed specifically for parents is a need currently unaddressed. The committee is proposing such a support group as a future project.

## COMMUNITY SUPPERS • Plainfield, NJ

The First Unitarian Society of Plainfield, in association with the Hyacinth Foundation, a community-based AIDS/HIV service organization in central New Jersey, sponsors monthly community suppers for people with AIDS/HIV and their partners, family members, and friends.

### Background and Development

Rev. Margaret Campbell-Gross, the minister of the Unitarian Society of Plainfield, proposed sponsoring a community supper program similar to one she participated in while ministering in San Francisco. The proposal met with quick and enthusiastic acceptance, and an AIDS subcommittee of the larger Outreach Committee formed to plan periodic meals for people with AIDS and their partners, family members, and friends.

Included in the initial planning was a representative of the Hyacinth Foundation, a nonprofit AIDS service organization based in New Jersey. This representative helped sensitize committee members to the multiple needs of people infected with AIDS. The committee membership quickly expanded to embrace all volunteers who wanted to contribute to this outreach effort, some of whom were not members of the church.

Beyond provision of healthy meals, planning committee members asked themselves, "What is the purpose of the community supper program?" Members did not want to focus on illness, and after conducting a community needs assessment, they learned that social and familial recreational opportunities were missing among the services available to people with AIDS. Thus, the purpose of the program emerged: to provide a comfortable and supportive environment in which people affected by AIDS might meet to enjoy good food, good company, good conversation, and a good time. The committee discovered that for some people with AIDS having a good time was an increasingly rare experience. These recreational meals would enable people with AIDS to feel fully human and cared for. Volunteers from both inside and outside the church joined the initial planners, and soon the committee put on the calendar the first of what are now monthly events.

Fifteen guests came to the first dinner in January 1990. These guests told other people affected by AIDS, and the number has since increased to between thirty-five and fifty at each meal.

*"One gains so much more than one gives. One gains in friendship and witness to the spirit of life. This is what church is all about. It's not a social club. It's a place for the whole congregation to refuel and to minister."*

**Rev. Margot Campbell-Gross**
**First Unitarian Society**
**Plainfield, NJ**

## Organization, Operation, and Resources

The committee began by widely distributing announcements. Area hospitals, gay and lesbian support groups, various AIDS support services, and methadone clinics sent flyers and assisted in their circulation. The coordinators of the program solicited RSVPs through a telephone number printed on the announcements. Because the number of responses received was never accurate, to estimate the size of a casserole and the number of places to be set became difficult. However, these problems were insignificant when weighed against the benefits of the program.

The supper program is now successfully serving a meal each month. The event begins at approximately 4:00 P.M. in the Steven's Room, a comfortable lounge in the church, with a social hour during which hors d'oeuvres and nonalcoholic beverages are served. At 5:00 P.M. people move into the parish hall for the buffet supper. The church provides a budget from which food is purchased for the suppers. Some food is also donated by members of the congregation. Those in charge of arranging the food cater to the special dietary needs of individual guests. For example, some persons with AIDS must restrict their intake of lactose, while others are vegetarian.

Volunteers are integral to the program. They help with publicity, food preparation, and decoration of the hall. Volunteers also perform live music at the gathering.

## BRUNCH PROGRAM • Brentwood, CA

Under the auspices of the Union of American Hebrew Congregations, members from synagogues in the Los Angeles area offer brunch to people with AIDS who come for treatment on an outpatient basis at the University of Southern California County Medical Center.

### Background and Development

Sharon Wahl, whose husband is a surgeon at the University of Southern California County Medical Center, discovered an acute problem in the Center's AIDS Outpatient Clinic, known as P521: patients in the twenty-bed hospital received three meals a day, but outpatients who came to P521 were given no food—even though they spent four to six hours waiting for treatment. The heaviest outpatient load came on Tuesdays and Thursdays. On Tuesdays, outpatients received blood infusions; on Thursdays they were given chemotherapy. No food was available for purchase in the clinic, and most of the outpatients had little money to buy food. Doctors told Wahl that the outpatients would receive chemotherapy treatment more comfortably if they had eaten a square meal that same day.

Wahl discussed this problem with members of her Sisterhood group at University Synagogue. Because Thursdays seemed to be the day of greatest need, the group organized brunch two Thursdays each month for outpatients at P521. Two additional synagogues—Leo Baeck Temple and Temple Isaiah—now offer brunch on the remaining Thursdays of each month, and Episcopal congregations have recently begun serving meals on Tuesdays.

### Organization, Operation, and Resources

Volunteers purchase food and meet at University Synagogue two Thursdays a month at 8:00 A.M. They then prepare the brunch, and those who do not have to leave for work bring the food to the Medical Center to begin serving by 10:30. Brunch ends around 2:00. The volunteers serve more than 200 egg salad and tuna salad sandwiches, potato and macaroni salad, juice, potato chips, and cookies. They provide food for 100 to 125 patients and staff each time they visit the clinic.

An extra benefit that the volunteers did not initially anticipate was that clients appreciate not only the food, but also the opportunity for conversation. For many, their hospital visit is the only social event in their lives.

Each brunch costs about $200. A Sisterhood fund designated for AIDS-related projects and the generous donations of the volunteers cover the cost. A few synagogue members have sponsored an entire brunch in memory of a loved one.

The majority of clients served are low-income people, from many walks of life, who have lost both their jobs and their insurance benefits.

## GOD'S LOVE WE DELIVER • New York, NY

The primary service of God's Love We Deliver is providing free healthy meals to homebound people with AIDS who are too debilitated by their illness to feed themselves. The ministry also coordinates a telephone networking system linking homebound people with AIDS to one another for mutual support and companionship.

### Background and Development

Ganga Stone founded God's Love We Deliver in 1985. As a hospice volunteer, Stone had delivered a bag of groceries to Richard, a young man confined to his home because of AIDS. Unemployed for over two years, Richard could not afford to order his meals and was too weak to prepare the food Stone had brought. Stone located Richard's friends and organized them to bring meals to him each day. This experience convinced Stone that an urgent need in the AIDS community was not being met.

Stone began cooking meals in her kitchen and delivering them on her bicycle with her friend Jane Ellen Best. Soon they enlisted the help of other volunteers. Early in 1986, Stone began what she called "Meals on Heels," which consisted of a core of volunteers picking up donated meals from approximately forty restaurants in New York City and delivering the meals on foot to clients in their area. The group quickly realized that the need for food exceeded the organization's ability to provide it.

In July 1987, the West Park Presbyterian Church in Manhattan donated its kitchen and a fourth-floor suite of offices and God's Love We Deliver thus became the first kitchen in New York City dedicated exclusively to feeding homebound people with AIDS. Project organizers conducted fund-raising events, recruited volunteers, and hired an executive chef. At its inception, God's Love We Deliver fed six homebound people. It has since grown and has served an estimated 140,000 meals to thousands of clients in its first five years of operation. Currently there are 350 active clients on its roster.

Expansion is moving ahead rapidly. Other kitchens have opened, one in the Bronx in the fall of 1990 at St. Peter's Episcopal Church and another in Brooklyn at St. Luke's and St. Matthew's. Other kitchens are planned for Queens and Washington, DC.

### Organization, Operation, and Resources

God's Love We Deliver is a community-based, nonprofit, secular organization of more than 650 active volunteers and a paid staff of thirty-two. Says Program Director Joan Block, "We deliver food, not sermons."

Cooking begins daily at 7:30 A.M. and meals go into four vans by 10:00 A.M., when work starts on the meals for the next day. By 2:30 P.M. everyone has been fed. The kitchen closes at 9:00 P.M.

*"If it weren't for God's Love, some days I wouldn't eat. If it weren't for these people, I wouldn't have gained back 10 to 15 pounds. They remember little things. They call me, hug me. It's very important for people in my situation. In 3 1/2 months, I gained 7 pounds from God's Love."*

On average, God's Love We Deliver provides nearly two hundred meals a day to clients in all five New York boroughs and Jersey City, New Jersey. Each meal consists of homemade soup; a green salad; a main course of meat, fish, or chicken; fresh vegetables; a carbohydrate; and dessert. The food is fresh, and the cooks make dishes from scratch, based on a rotating thirty-day menu. The foods are high calorie, low microbe, and high protein as recommended by nutritionists for people with AIDS. The menu includes dishes such as carrot bisque, artichoke salad, smoked turkey, four-cheese lasagna, veal stroganoff, marinated bean salad, a kabob of chicken with mushrooms and peppers on saffron rice, freshly baked cookies, pears in puff pastry, and fruit Bavarian.

Volunteers pack the meals in temperature-controlled storage containers and transport them by van to individuals in need or to drop-off centers. Much of the work of God's Love We Deliver comes from its dedicated corps of volunteers who prepare and deliver the meals. Interns from area colleges also work for the program, and a small number of young people from England volunteer during the summer months.

A partnership has developed between God's Love We Deliver and local communities of faith. The program director and volunteer coordinator reach out to churches and synagogues, and a large pool of volunteers have come from these communities. Volunteers are trained and enter a position best suited to their interests and time commitments.

Churches and synagogues, along with businesses, also serve as distribution drop-off centers. Volunteers deliver meals to these sites and other volunteers pick up the meals and take them to clients in their own neighborhoods.

The approximate cost of meals per week, per client, is $20. Cash and donations from individuals and organizations help defray expenses and restaurants supply supplemental meals when required. Celebrity fund-raisers have successfully brought in additional revenues. A very small percentage of the program's yearly budget comes from government grants.

The office of the New York mayor, David Dinkins, appropriated funds for a new van, and former mayor Ed Koch provided a city-owned van for the organization's use. Department stores and other businesses and organizations have also been generous. For example, Bloomingdales provided the ministry with all its stainless steel cookware and a food processor. For a Thanksgiving dinner, the store roasted and donated 500 pounds of turkey and made a $4,000 contribution. The New York City Gay Men's Chorus donated a giant walk-in refrigerator.

Individuals also contribute to the effort. For example, an upper West Side florist donates flowers, which help bring extra cheer to holiday meals. Another individual donated a computer to monitor the organization's operations.

# FOOD & FRIENDS • Washington, DC

Food & Friends is a nonprofit community organization with a mission to provide nutritious meals and human caring to homebound people with AIDS who are too ill and impoverished to provide adequate food for themselves.

## Background and Development

In May 1989, Food & Friends opened a kitchen in space donated by Westminster Presbyterian Church in southwest Washington, DC. The church was responding to "AIDS in Light of the Gospel," a resolution by the Presbyterian Church's Committee on Social Witness Policy. One section of this document specifically states that "presbyteries and congregations should use their human and material resources to respond to the AIDS crisis with support groups, counseling, grants, facilities for recreational activities, and community organization of persons with AIDS."

## Organization, Operation, and Resources

Food & Friends provides eight-course meals delivered at midday Monday through Friday. These meals provide 100 percent of the recommended daily allowance for nutrients and calories. The meals include homemade soups, fresh salads, entrees, desserts, and a light breakfast for the next day. The group tailors special meals to meet the needs of individuals with dietary restrictions. Examples of menu items include vegetable bisque, tomato chickpea salad with Dijon vinaigrette, perch Florentine, carrots and herbs, sage onion bread, white rice, and chocolate puff.

Volunteers help cook and package the food under the supervision of a professional chef, who has expertise in nutrition, menu planning, the preparation of large quantities of freshly cooked foods, safety and sanitary requirements, and the purchasing of food and kitchen supplies.

A driver transports the meals at midday in thermal containers to individual clients and families or to drop-off centers located throughout the District of Columbia and sections of Maryland and Virginia. Other volunteers pick up meals from centers in neighborhoods where they live or work and deliver the meals to clients.

The staff includes an executive director, the chef, a services coordinator, a volunteer coordinator, and a delivery driver. A corps of 100 volunteers help in the kitchen and office, deliver meals, and assist with fund-raising events.

Volunteers are young and old, of all ethnic and racial backgrounds, religious and nonreligious. Students from five inner-city and suburban high schools earn academic credit for community service by volunteering for Food & Friends. College, seminary, and university students deliver meals between classes. The group has recruited volunteers from churches, Retired Seniors Volunteer Program (RSVP), the Kiwanis Club, and court probation

*"The value of what I owe Food & Friends is incalculable. What I received from chopping vegetables, stirring soup, and washing pots and pans was a much-needed perspective: my vague disgruntlement with life paled beside individuals facing the end of their life. I also received a sense of immediacy and satisfaction rare in my field of history. The value of what I do professionally is unclear for years. At Food & Friends, the food I helped prepare at ten o'clock sustained someone at noon. That's tangible gratification!"*

**Keep in mind that food drives can be successfully extended to non-food items as well. Toothpaste, soap, shaving cream—these goods are always appreciated by homebound PWAs and their families.**

officers who recommend community service. Drop-off centers established by Food & Friends enable people who work full-time to participate by delivering meals during their lunch hour near their work place.

## YOM RISHON AIDS FOOD DRIVE • Washington, DC

The Yom Rishon AIDS Food Drive, a project of the Washington Committee of the National Jewish AIDS Project, coordinates the collection of nonperishable food items from synagogues in the Washington, DC, area and delivers this food to the AIDS Food Bank of the Whitman-Walker Clinic.

### Background and Development

The National Jewish AIDS Project was founded in 1986 to provide AIDS education programs in the Jewish community on the local and national level and to raise funds to assist organizations providing services to persons with AIDS.

The Washington Committee of the National Jewish AIDS Project held evening fund-raisers to channel funds from the local Jewish community to the Whitman-Walker Clinic. Committee members searched for a program idea involving more people while serving as a consciousness raiser and educational tool on AIDS issues. After discussion, the members agreed to sponsor a food bank. To coordinate the project, the director and chair of the Washington Committee brought together a number of volunteers who were members of local synagogues or who volunteered with the Whitman-Walker Clinic.

The committee agreed on the name Yom Rishon (literally "one Sunday" in Hebrew) AIDS Food Drive, printed stationery, and sent letters and brochures to every synagogue in the Washington, DC, area (including the suburbs of Maryland and Virginia). The letter, sent to the rabbi, the president, and the chair of each synagogue's social action committee, explained the concept of the project. The brochure provided a suggested list of food items that were especially needed for the food bank. The Washington Committee asked synagogue officials to return an enclosed form to the National Jewish AIDS Project pledging their willingness to participate in the food drive. The committee followed the letter with a phone call.

The Food Bank of the Whitman-Walker Clinic was opened in 1988 to provide basic food items at no cost to people living with AIDS.

### Organization, Operation, and Resources

The Washington Committee assigns each synagogue that wishes to participate in this food drive a one-month time slot and asks the synagogue to choose one Sunday in that month. Each of the forty participating synagogues picks one Sunday and asks its congregants to bring nonperishable food items to the synagogue on or before that day. Volunteers from the Washington Committee and from the Whitman-Walker Clinic collect the food at the synagogue and deliver it to the food bank.

Each synagogue advertises its Yom Rishon Day through newsletters, mailings, and announcements. Many divert their existing food drives to AIDS for the given month. To promote the food drive, some synagogues include speakers at services and educational programs geared to teens and children. At some Hebrew schools, teachers make the food drive a classroom project and children color grocery bags and write messages to persons with AIDS.

Since the start of the food drive, three synagogues have donated food they received during Kol Nidre—an October night when almost every congregant attends services and donates food. One synagogue has volunteered to do three food drives. Another mailed notices to all its members and received 200 bags of food in one day.

The Food Bank of the Whitman-Walker Clinic stocks tuna, canned soup and vegetables, pasta, peanut butter, instant milk, baby food, toothpaste, facial tissues, shaving cream, and other nonperishable food and personal items.

*"I don't always have the strength or energy to cook, but I look forward to superb meals every day. After my third surgery I weighed 98 pounds. Now I weigh 120. The meals help ease my mom's worry. She can't be home much because she works two jobs. Having the meals provided and having a friend stop by and check on me gets me through."*

## PROJECT OPEN HAND • San Francisco, CA

Project Open Hand is a meal-service program that provides hot, nutritious meals to homebound people with AIDS or ARC who are too weak or too impoverished to care for themselves.

### Background and Development

Ruth Brinker founded Project Open Hand in 1985, after experiencing the death of a close friend who had AIDS. While Brinker and a few others provided meals for their friend when he became too weak to prepare food for himself, Brinker worried about other homebound people with AIDS who did not have this care and support. After making numerous phone calls, Brinker was given a list of seven people with AIDS who needed assistance. Within a month, the number rose to thirty-five. After five years, Open Hand, the only organization of its kind in the San Francisco Bay area, fed more than fifteen hundred clients a day.

Currently, Open Hand has fifty-two full-time employees and operates with the support of nearly one thousand community volunteers who prepare and deliver the meals each day.

## Organization, Operation, and Resources

Because many people with AIDS were suffering not only from the effects of the virus but also from malnutrition, Ruth Brinker began Open Hand with the conviction that the project should offer meals to anyone who needed them, regardless of the person's ability to pay, and would use only the highest quality foods. To date, only 15 percent of Open Hand's clients can afford the daily donation for their meals.

Volunteers prepare meals from scratch using fresh ingredients with all necessary nutrients, including the nine trace elements nutritionists suggest for people with AIDS. The project requests a letter of diagnosis within a two-week period after service has begun.

Churches, synagogues, and businesses serve as drop-off centers where parishioners and other volunteers pick up meals and deliver them to clients in their own neighborhoods, either on foot or in pairs. (One person could drive while the other could act as a "runner," delivering meals to a client's door.)

Open Hand's volunteers come from all walks of life. Some young people donate a few hours a week after school and on weekends; some retirees and working people donate time each day to the project. Other helpers perform court-mandated community service at Open Hand. Celebrities, such as Shirley MacLaine, have produced thirty-second public service announcements that have aired on local television and radio stations. These announcements inform the community of Open Hand's services and help recruit volunteers.

Operational monies come from foundations, corporations, direct-mail donors, special events, bequests, estates, and other sources. Less than one percent of Open Hand's funding comes from government agencies. The Open Hand's kitchen is a 3,800-square-foot state-of-the-art facility paid for by foundation grants.

Open Hand primarily serves people in San Francisco. However, the organization has been able to offer hot meal services on a part-time basis to some people with AIDS in the hard-hit Alameda County area, east of San Francisco. Attempts are currently underway to solicit funds that will enable the project to offer its services on a full-time basis to the increasing number of people with AIDS living in the East Bay Area.

The program's evaluation process is simple: as long as each client receives a good, well-balanced meal each day, the organization's mission and goals are being accomplished. Over the past five years, the organization has never missed serving a single meal to a client who requested food—even during the project's move to a new facility and during the devastating earthquake that hit the Bay Area in October of 1989.

## OPEN HAND CHICAGO • Chicago, IL

Open Hand provides meals across the city of Chicago to people with AIDS and ARC and their dependents.

### Background and Development

Following the Chicago NAMES Project Quilt display in July 1988, a group of volunteers met to discuss what practical help they could provide to people with AIDS/ARC in Chicago. They realized that grocery shopping and preparing food can be difficult for persons with AIDS/ARC and that providing meals would make a real difference in the quality of these individuals' lives.

Modeled after Project Open Hand, the successful San Francisco program, Open Hand Chicago began meal delivery on January 2, 1989.

### Organization, Operation, and Resources

Volunteers for Open Hand Chicago deliver two meals, one hot and one "brown bag," seven days a week to people with AIDS/ARC and to members of their households. Volunteers prepare meals using fresh, high-quality ingredients. Open Hand Chicago works with a nutritionist to meet the dietary needs of all its clients.

Community agencies, physicians, and hospitals refer clients, or clients call on their own and ask for meals. As part of the sign-up process, a nutritional assessment is performed. In designing a meal, the organization pays attention to the client's medical condition (diet prescribed, medications taken, infections present) and personal preferences (favorite foods, religious restrictions).

Food and supplies are donated or purchased, and volunteers prepare and package approximately two hundred meals a day, Monday through Friday, at a central location. A team of volunteer drivers and runners (those who take the food from the car into the house or apartment building) deliver the meals. The "runner" provides support to the client and can determine if the client is in need of immediate health care.

Volunteers also help with office work (data entry, filing, phones), produce the volunteer newsletter, conduct fund-raising events, and help in public relations efforts. Volunteers include clergy, seniors, gay men, lesbians, bisexual people, students, homemakers, and business people. Some volunteers are people with AIDS who work in all aspects of the organization. Volunteers hear about the program through announcements in the gay and mainstream press and in presentations given by the staff of Open Hand Chicago in churches, synagogues, and schools. College and high school seniors serve as interns and receive school credit for their involvement in the project.

The owners at Thorek Hospital have donated their kitchen to the project for food preparation and packaging. Food packages, which are free to all

*"I have just been given eight weeks to live. This monumental problem, in addition to the 'normal' problems of AIDS, made the work of Open Hand very timely. It came when despair had just started to creep into my life."*

*"After my nephew became sick, I felt I needed to do something so that another person would not be abandoned. Taking food to somebody is just a little way of helping."*

clients, cost an average of $3.50 each. Funds for this come from fund-raising events, individual and group donations, bequests, and corporate grants. National corporations, such as Sara Lee and Xerox, as well as members of the Chicago business community, have donated to the project. Donations have included kitchen appliances, office equipment, computers, and typewriters.

Project organizers hope to expand the operation by purchasing a "satellite" kitchen in another area of the city.

# Housing and Hospices

*"One does not love a place less for having suffered in it."*
—Jane Austen

## DEWOLFE HOUSE • Seattle, WA

The AIDS Housing Project of the University Unitarian Church in Seattle, Washington, in association with the Northwest AIDS Foundation, sponsors the DeWolfe House, an independent-living residence for men with AIDS.

### Background and Development

In 1987, the minister at the University Unitarian Church gave a sermon on the need for people to get involved in a compassionate response to AIDS. Some members of the congregation decided to organize a group to look into the possibility of starting a project related to AIDS. They contacted the Northwest AIDS Foundation, their local AIDS service organization, to determine which services were in high demand. The group (by that time known as the UUC AIDS Task Force) discovered that though housing was available for people with AIDS who were in the final stages of the illness, little was available for those who could live independently but lacked sufficient financial resources. The AIDS Housing Project, a subgroup of the UUC AIDS Task Force, grew out of this need.

In November 1987, members of the AIDS Housing Project chose to focus on meeting the housing needs of persons with AIDS in the King County area. Congregation members donated $30,000, including a $10,000 "matching grant" donated anonymously by one individual, to purchase a house. Additional donations came from the Seattle Foundation, from the Seattle Men's Chorus, and from Unitarian churches nationwide.

In August 1988, the AIDS Housing Project opened the DeWolfe House, named to honor the memory of Rev. Mark Mosher DeWolfe, a Unitarian Universalist minister who died of AIDS in July 1988.

### Organization, Operation, and Resources

The DeWolfe House is organized as a residence for men with AIDS who are capable of living independently, but who are financially unable to remain in their own homes. The house is a seven-bedroom, two-story residence, situated in a neighborhood with other group-living houses near health facilities in the Capitol Hill section of Seattle. Residents share common living areas and have their own private bedrooms. The AIDS Housing Project provides a

*"University Unitarian Church's fifth-grade class arranged a special visit with the residents of DeWolfe House. The students prepared a spectacular brunch of omelettes, fruit, and muffins. What struck many of the students most strongly was how the residents all seemed just like nice 'normal' guys. The kids confirmed that DeWolfe House is fulfilling its purpose of allowing people with AIDS to live as normal a life as possible."*

DeWolfe House News

When starting a residential program, develop clear policy guidelines that outline behaviors considered unacceptable (especially with regard to substance abuse). Detail how the program will deal with violations of the guidelines.

bed and chest of drawers for each bedroom.

The residents are responsible for buying and preparing their own food, managing their own money, and maintaining personal hygiene. A resident advocate and individual case managers who coordinate social services for the residents provide referral and advocacy services.

The University Unitarian Church owns the home and is responsible for its maintenance. The church charges residents a low monthly rent and keeps open rooms for them during short periods of inpatient hospital care. The Northwest AIDS Foundation administers the selection of residents and is one of many care providers with whom the University Unitarian Church works to ensure that the health care and social service needs of the residents are met.

To become a resident at DeWolfe House a person must be a citizen of King County, Washington; establish financial need; be able to pay the monthly rent of $125 (this requirement can be waived if a person is critically disabled by HIV infection); provide certification by a licensed physician that he has AIDS; indicate willingness and ability to live cooperatively in a group situation; be able to live independently; be free from drug and alcohol dependency or be willing to enter a treatment program if that is recommended after an evaluation by a substance-abuse counselor; be willing to make out a will to ensure the rightful handling of personal property; sign an admission agreement prior to acceptance; sign release forms permitting the case manager and staff to obtain medical and psychological information as needed to develop a plan of care and coordinate appropriate services; supply references from previous landlords and personal references; and agree to work with a case manager and the residence advisor to coordinate services and assure financial assistance.

Residents attend weekly house meetings in which they discuss organizational and housekeeping issues and problems related to community living.

Because of the ever-present possibility of discrimination, the address and phone number of the residence remains private and confidential. All persons involved with the residence—residents, friends of residents, volunteers, and paid care providers—agree to maintain confidentiality.

Volunteers help with the restoration and maintenance of the DeWolfe House and assist residents with daily needs. One volunteer, a retired architect, fixes the plumbing when problems arise, assists with yard work, waits around the house for the gas and phone companies to come, and accepts deliveries.

## CLUSTER HOUSING—THE PLYMOUTH MODEL • Seattle, WA

Plymouth Congregational Church subsidizes and equips "cluster housing" in the Seattle area for low-income persons with AIDS who wish to live independently. Cluster housing meets the needs of people who want neither the closeness of a group home nor the isolation of a single apartment. By living in a cluster of apartments all located in one building, they can be on their own and still enjoy the benefits of a caring and attentive community.

This Project received a Special Project Award for Distinguished and Exemplary Service in AIDS/HIV Ministry from the AIDS National Interfaith Network in 1990.

### Background and Development

In 1987, Seattle's AIDS service community estimated that an increasing number of persons with AIDS required housing assistance. By 1990 the Northwest AIDS Foundation expected that more than half its clients would need help with housing because nearly three-quarters of them earned less than $400 a month. In 1988, the Seattle Housing Authority agreed to set aside twenty low-income units in sites scattered throughout the city. The Northwest AIDS Foundation established a rent-subsidy account to funnel donations from churches and other sources on an emergency basis to those in need.

What was not available, however, was long-term housing for clients who preferred to remain independent but could no longer afford to stay in market-rate housing. The 1,100-member Plymouth congregation responded by offering to subsidize and furnish studio apartments in a downtown Seattle apartment building (The Payne Apartments) near medical and social services. Tenants would pay half the real rent per month, which the subsidy account would then match. A group of Plymouth church members established the Plymouth Housing Group to oversee this project.

The Plymouth Housing Group, which functions as the Payne landlord, opened the restored forty-five-unit Payne Apartments in June 1988 to provide affordable housing for persons of low income. The Plymouth Housing Group reserved a cluster of four studio apartments at the Payne for people living with AIDS and furnished them through donations from members and friends of the church. The group used a gift of $500 to reestablish telephone service to each of the units. Through its mission budget, Plymouth also subsidized these units with a monthly donation of $300. With the addition of two units in 1990, the Housing Group now subsidizes six apartments. By 1991, these units had been home to at least two dozen persons with AIDS.

If you begin a project like this, make an inventory of the furniture on loan to the tenants. Also, make the rooms as appealing as possible. Welcome each new tenant with a clean, orderly room, because tenants take better care of a place that looks good when they move in. Reward tenants who prove to be responsible and who want to improve their room by upgrading their furniture and equipment as these are donated. As long as rooms pass a monthly inspection, leave the tenants in peace.

**This type of project requires not only minimal financial investment but also minimal volunteer power. A handful of volunteers maintain the apartments between tenants and pick up donated furniture. (Donating furniture is also an easy way for people to get involved.)**

## Organization, Operation, and Resources

For tenants with AIDS, living at the Payne is much like living in any other low-income apartment building. Residents cook their own meals, do their own laundry, and experience the occasional frustrations of leaky plumbing or temperamental heat. Each unit has a main room, walk-in closet, separate kitchen, and separate bath. The rent includes all utilities, except telephone and cable television.

The Northwest AIDS Foundation identifies and refers prospective tenants with AIDS to the landlord and assures that the tenants are linked through a case manager to appropriate services. At the Payne the manager screens prospective tenants just as any apartment manager would. All tenants must abide by common building rules—from paying their portion of the rent on time to keeping peace with their neighbors.

AIDS tenants in the Plymouth program vary from those who have always been low-income to those whose economic status has fallen because of AIDS. Most are gay men in their twenties; some are able to work and/or attend school, most maintain active social lives. The AIDS tenants stay from one month to two or more years. The most common reason for leaving is inability to manage finances for timely payment of rent. Like other tenants in the building, a few have been evicted for drug dealing or disruptive behavior.

Informal monthly meetings give the AIDS tenants the opportunity to check in with one another and to voice their concerns. In attendance at these meetings are the tenants, the Northwest AIDS Foundation's housing advocate assigned to the Payne, the building manager and assistant, and the Plymouth coordinator.

Plymouth furnishes and equips the six apartments set aside for people with AIDS to match the needs of each tenant as closely as possible. Some tenants need to be loaned furniture for the entire apartment; others arrive with ample personal belongings and want no set up. Plymouth loans furniture and equipment to the tenants, with the understanding that most everything will be left behind when they move. Because many items "walked away" early in the project, project directors make an inventory of each unit, and the Foundation holds the tenant accountable for missing major items. Plymouth maintains a storeroom for donated items.

One Plymouth volunteer organizes cleaning after each tenant leaves. Cleaning is easy if the previous tenant has left the unit in rent-ready condition. If not, additional volunteers help, and the Payne manager makes repairs and repaints as necessary. One volunteer ascertains from the Foundation or from the Payne staff what the new tenant is likely to want in the apartment. Once the tenant has moved in, that volunteer is back in contact to see if anything else is needed.

The church newsletter and Sunday morning announcements keep the Plymouth members updated on the AIDS project. Such communication also nets needed items not already on hand. The Plymouth Housing Group offers surplus items to the Payne manager for other tenants in the building or to other housing projects and sells unusable items to keep cash available for incidental purchases. Donors bring items directly to the Payne or call for a pickup by a Plymouth volunteer. The church provides a tax receipt, when requested, and refers inappropriate items to other agencies that might be interested in them.

## THE AIDS LODGING HOUSE • Portland, ME

The AIDS Lodging House provides affordable housing in a safe, homelike environment for persons with AIDS/HIV. Four furnished apartments are available for a small rental fee, which includes utilities, phone, cable television, and light housekeeping services.

The Lodging House, which was formed to assist persons with AIDS who must live on low incomes, is located in Portland (Maine's largest city) near several major medical facilities. The house is open to any and all persons with AIDS from Maine who are over eighteen years of age and who can live independently and cooperatively with others in a communal setting.

### Background and Development

The AIDS Lodging House was founded and incorporated in 1987 by a diverse group from the Portland area concerned that many people living with AIDS/HIV were unable to find safe and affordable housing. Dr. Michael Bach, a local physician treating many persons with AIDS/HIV in the Portland area, was the first to alert the community to the need for such housing. After much preparatory work, a four-unit apartment building was purchased in 1988 as a lodging house and two apartments were opened in the spring of 1989. As remodeling was finished, two more units became available. A total of seven residents now occupy the house.

### Organization, Operation, and Resources

The Lodging House is a large duplex, with several communal kitchens and living areas. Each resident has his or her own bedroom. Also available are a backyard and garden area. The house is within close proximity to hospitals, social services, and the downtown area. It provides a supportive atmosphere for independent living in which residents can plan and provide for their own needs. The house is fully equipped and furnished, but residents who wish to use their own bedroom furnishings may bring what fits comfortably in their rooms.

What makes the group housing concept especially challenging is that the independence that attracts a person living with AIDS to such a home is also the independence that prompts a person who is dying to resist moving to more appropriate housing. The telephone becomes a critical link, as does a pass key for care givers. Sadly, you must sometimes be willing to let the person die alone.

**Be particular about the location of your low-income housing. While convenient to many services for tenants with AIDS, a downtown location also means the tenants have limited sources of affordable groceries, toiletries, and household items. Also, drug dealing and other illegal activities may be too close for comfort. Screen out prospective tenants for whom such ready temptation would jeopardize successful placement.**

The AIDS Lodging House is an independent agency with its own board of directors. The Maine State Housing Authority funds the project. A grant from the State of Maine through the Department of Human Services meets the administrative and personnel costs. Churches, businesses, and individuals donate other funds and furnishings. A salaried program director runs the Lodging House, and volunteers assist on a needed basis, doing painting and other maintenance work.

Applicants must sign an Admissions Agreement and Liability Release Form. Because of the communal nature of the project, they must abide by house rules listed in the "Lodging House Policy and Procedures Manual," which they are given prior to residency. Lodgers must also agree to a statement of confidentiality. That is, no person involved in Lodging House— a resident, a friend or a family member of a resident, a volunteer, or a paid staff or provider—is to discuss other residents with people not involved in the Lodging House. In addition, the address and phone number of the Lodging House are considered confidential.

The first thirty days of residence in the Lodging House are a probationary period during which time either the resident or the Lodging House can negate the terms of the Admissions Agreement.

Residents must attend weekly house meetings. During the first part of the meeting, residents discuss business issues. During the second part a group leader, other than the house manager, facilitates a discussion in which the residents share feelings, give emotional support, and explore issues of communal living.

## SAVE, INC. • Kansas City, MO

The SAVE Home is an AIDS hospice in Kansas City, Missouri.

### Background and Development

In the spring of 1986, members of the Kansas City business community met to discuss what to do on a local level to help people with AIDS. As a result, they established the SAVE Foundation to provide assistance to people with AIDS who lack alternative resources.

### Organization, Operation, and Resources

The SAVE Home, the only AIDS hospice in Missouri, is a residential home with six private bedrooms. Residents share a common living room, dining room, and kitchen. Currently a full-time housing director, assistant director, and three full-time paid staff members run the home and provide twenty-four-hour care. With the assistance of volunteers, staff members schedule services for residents, clean the house, prepare meals, and administer patient care. Under the guidance of St. Mark's Union Church, the housing director supervises the residences.

Most residents come from the Kansas City area, though the home has no residential requirements. Residents range in age from the early twenties to the middle fifties. Due to illness, these residents have no other housing alternatives.

Social service agencies and physicians refer applicants. Upon acceptance, a resident signs a contract agreeing to follow house policies. As long as the residents abide by the contract, they may remain at the home as long as needed.

The SAVE Foundation, which sponsors the home, is an independent, nonprofit foundation, funded in significant part by private contributions. Individuals donate money, household goods, furniture, and time. Community organizations lend support by helping to sponsor fund-raising events.

*"The residences are places to live—not hospitals. SAVE residents enjoy the companionship and shared strength of people in similar circumstances."*

**A SAVE Foundation brochure**

## PETER CLAVER COMMUNITY • San Francisco, CA

The Peter Claver Community provides long-term housing and comprehensive support services to thirty-two homeless men and women with AIDS/ARC.

### Background and Development

In 1985, the San Francisco Department of Public Health convened the first meeting of the Mayor's Task Force on housing for persons with AIDS/ARC who were homeless because of substance abuse, neurological impairments, and/or behavioral problems that made them ineligible for other existing forms of housing.

The consortium included individuals from various AIDS service organizations, medical facilities, and government agencies who were concerned with meeting the needs of the ever-increasing population of homeless persons with AIDS/ARC.

Within a year and a half, the Department of Public Health allocated funds to initiate a new program, and officials asked Catholic Charities of San Francisco to begin a residential program to serve this homeless population.

The AIDS/ARC Residential Program (now known as the Peter Claver Community) began in March 1987 to provide long-term housing and on-site support services (case management, counseling, money management, client advocacy) to thirty-two homeless men and women with AIDS or ARC. Through a generous contribution and additional government subsidies, the

**You may find it necessary to evict drug users for nonpayment of rent. Frequently they leave behind disheveled rooms, where syringes are easily concealed. Instruct volunteers who clean the rooms to beware of syringes and to dispose of them in a sharps container (a safe receptacle with a one-way door).**

program relocated to its new site in August 1988.

### Organization, Operation, and Resources

The Peter Claver Community is named after a missionary who ministered to slaves in the New World by offering them food, medical attention, and spiritual support. A director, an assistant director/case manager, two case managers, a money manager/case manager, a volunteer coordinator/case manager, an adult day-care coordinator, a part-time psychiatric nurse, an administrative assistant, and four overnight paraprofessional staff members staff this residential program. The building management staff, which is contracted independently, includes a building administrator, full-time janitorial and maintenance service, and twenty-four-hour desk clerk coverage. In addition, four hours per week of consultation from a psychiatrist working for the AIDS Health Project is available to the program.

The program, which provides long-term housing, permits residents to stay throughout the progression of their illness, if attendant care providers can adequately care for them. The social services staff provides client advocacy, counseling, psychosocial assessment, case management, and coordination of treatment plans. Catholic Charities receives the clients' welfare benefits, deducts one-third to cover housing fees, and gives the client the balance.

The Visiting Nurse Hospice Program and other home health care agencies assess in-house support services and attendant care. The assigned case manager arranges psychiatric assessment and consultation as needed for the residents. The adult day-care component offers art therapy, creative writing, a therapeutic swim program, and weekend activities or outings. Project Open Hand furnishes lunch and dinner. Weekly on-site Narcotics Anonymous, Alcoholics Anonymous, and early recovery meetings are also available for the residents.

The volunteer coordinator recruits by announcing the program in local gay and mainstream newspapers, and Catholic Charities reaches out to area parishes. Volunteers, who provide emotional and practical support and assist with adult day-care activities, teach swimming, art, cooking, and massage; facilitate workshops; and help clean the home. Besides being available for outings into the community, they also provide residents with transportation to and from appointments. All volunteers must attend a daylong training at Peter Claver that addresses topics such as AIDS, substance abuse, codependency, and skills for setting limits.

Funding for the program comes from the San Francisco Department of Public Health's Medically Indigent Adult Program and the City's Division of Mental Health, Substance Abuse, and Forensics. Support also comes from individuals.

## ST. ANTHONY'S HOME • Baton Rouge, LA

The Baton Rouge AIDS Task Force sponsors St. Anthony's Home, a living program for people with AIDS. Our Lady of the Lake Regional Medical Center's Immunological Support Group manages the home, which serves persons who are indigent because of AIDS.

### Background and Development

In 1987, it became clear to many concerned citizens in the Baton Rouge area that there was a desperate need for safe and affordable housing for persons living with AIDS/HIV. A vacant house was donated to Our Lady of the Lake Regional Medical Center and is used for the project. A local interior decorator's group sponsored the renovations and donated supplies and furnishings. A landscaping company also donated its services. The home opened in January 1988.

### Organization, Operation, and Resources

St. Anthony's Home can accommodate seven residents. To become a resident of St. Anthony's Home, a person must be diagnosed with AIDS, be in need of a place to live, be eighteen years of age or older, and be able and willing to live in a group setting.

Residents share a furnished bedroom with one other person. Around-the-clock staff are available to assist residents. The cost to each resident is fifty percent of his or her monthly income or $300, whichever is smaller. The cost includes meals. Volunteers, who come from the local AIDS Task Force, help with recreational activities, lawn care, meals, and periodic house repairs and transport residents to medical appointments.

Funding for the home, including staff salaries, comes from Our Lady of the Lake Regional Medical Center and from private donations. Donations from individuals and community groups provide medication and incidental expenses for each resident. Various church and professional groups donate meals on a designated schedule, and the local food bank donates some food staples. A federal housing grant covers additional operating expenses.

*"We've worked to create a sense of family. St. Anthony's is a home, and it in no way resembles a hospital. Some people have said it's the nicest home they've ever had."*

**Ken McLeod**
**Manager**
**St. Anthony's Home**

## ADOPT-A-ROOM • Boston, MA

The Adopt-A-Room project of the Interfaith Assembly on Homelessness and Housing brings together religious and community groups to contribute in the furnishing of residences for homeless people. Though not specifically an AIDS-related project, the Adopt-A-Room concept can be duplicated to provide furnished housing for homeless people with AIDS/HIV.

**To assess the needs of your tenants, schedule regular tenant meetings and informal encounters.**

## Background and Development

In October 1986, the Social Action Ministries and the Jewish Community Relations Council of Greater Boston sponsored a press conference to address the housing and homelessness crisis. This union resulted in the creation of the Interfaith Assembly on Homelessness and Housing (IAHH), which is modeled after a successful New York City program. Clergy and lay leaders of many faiths organized IAHH.

## Organization, Operation, and Resources

The Adopt-A-Room project organizes community groups, congregations, and individuals in an effort to donate cash or furnishings to complete the development of a room for homeless people in a permanent residence. The specific objectives of the Adopt-A-Room project are the following: to furnish and decorate rooms for homeless people in permanent affordable housing units; to empower homeless women and men to take charge of their lives while preserving their human dignity and self-respect; to provide an opportunity for participants to make a direct and meaningful contribution to the effort to house the homeless; and to enable even small investors to make a tangible difference in the lives of homeless women and men, thereby encouraging their continuing commitment to solve the problem of homelessness.

An adopting group contacts IAHH and chooses the type of room to adopt. IAHH pairs groups with housing for the homeless built by nonprofit developers. IAHH sends the adopting group a description of the room and the furnishings they need to acquire. IAHH asks adopting groups to donate furniture or the estimated costs of furnishing a room. For instance, a bedroom furnished with a bed, desk, bureau, chairs, lamps, curtains, pictures, mirror, clock radio, linens, blankets, and pillows costs $800; a dining room furnished with dining room table, chairs, buffet, table linens, lamps, pictures, and curtains costs $700; a living room furnished with a sofa, stuffed chairs, tables, lamps, television, pictures, and curtains costs $1,000; a kitchen costs $300 for appliances, pots and pans, utensils, dishes, curtains, clock, and flatware; and miscellaneous rooms and spaces (halls, bathrooms, gardens) cost between $50 and $250.

Three to six months may elapse between the initial commitment to adopt and the actual furnishing of a room. Adopting groups use this period to raise funds or acquire high-quality used furniture from their congregations or membership. IAHH facilitates cash contributions in lieu of furniture purchases and schedules a day for the adopting groups and other volunteers to deliver furniture and decorate the rooms. The room adopters can join with the developers and the new tenants to celebrate the opening of the new housing.

# Drop-In and Day-Care Centers

"One word frees us of all the weight and pain of life: that word is love."
—Sophocles

## FRANCIS HOUSE • Tampa, FL

Francis House is an interfaith drop-in center for people affected by HIV. It is dedicated to St. Francis of Assisi, whose love for all people as sisters and brothers inspires its staff and volunteers. Until project coordinators purchase a space, services are provided at St. Paul Lutheran Church in Tampa, Florida.

### Background and Development

Francis House was developed out of a spiritual support group in July 1989. Sister Anne Dougherty provided much of the leadership for the project following the death of a friend to AIDS one year earlier.

### Organization, Operation, and Resources

Services at this drop-in center (which has a relaxed and homey atmosphere) include individual and group counseling; art, music, and movement therapy; and group meditation. Francis House offers its ongoing programs both day and night. Volunteers facilitate these programs. Francis House coordinates many programs with the Tampa AIDS Network and the People with AIDS Coalition. Private donations, churches, and grants provide the funding. One full-time staff person coordinates the project.

*"Trust in God and have your roots deep in spirituality. If your program is of God, it will happen."*

**Sister Anne Dougherty**
**Director**
**Francis House**

## PASTORAL CARE AT THE WELLNESS CENTER AT PACKARD MANSE • Stoughton, MA

The drop-in center for persons living with AIDS/HIV at Packard Manse includes a food pantry, short-term counseling, noon meals and snacks, potluck dinners, a coffee house, and pastoral care.

### Background and Development

A coalition of religious, health, holistic, volunteer, professional, and community-based groups joined those at Packard Manse in January 1990 to

*"There is a special spirit I feel when I come to the Manse. I can be myself. I feel accepted. It's a place to relax, talk, listen to music, read, and share a meal with people who care about me as a person."*

establish the Wellness Center for all affected by HIV.

## Organization, Operation, and Resources

A pastoral care coordinator runs the drop-in center at Packard Manse, which is open two days a week. The goal is to be open every weekday. Volunteers are the sole staff.

The volunteers plan a potluck dinner for the first Tuesday and a coffee house for the third Friday of every month. At the coffee house, the volunteers provide live entertainment, music, special teas and coffees, pastries, and conversation. Volunteer assistance is given both on and off the premises with transportation, shopping, errands, respite care, and household help.

The center depends entirely on donations gathered from individuals and from various fund-raising activities. The fund-raising and steering committees meet once a month to plan and strategize.

## HERO DROP-IN CENTER • Baltimore, MD

The Health Education Resource Organization (HERO) provides a drop-in center for people with HIV disease and AIDS in a space donated by the congregations of St. John's United Methodist Church and the Metropolitan Community Church of Baltimore. The center offers lunch and provides recreation, entertainment, arts and crafts, and free services, such as haircuts and massage. The center is free to all clients.

### Background and Development

Operating since 1983, HERO is Maryland's largest AIDS-service provider. HERO offers education and outreach prevention, operates the Maryland State AIDS Hotline, has an extensive educational materials department, and provides direct client services to any HIV-infected person. As the organization grew during the 1980s, many clients expressed a need for a common area where they could go during the day for support and recreation.

In 1990, Indira Kotval, HERO's Administrator for Client Services, visited drop-in centers for people with AIDS/HIV in San Francisco and New York to get ideas for a similar project proposed in Maryland. For months, HERO searched for an inexpensive space that it could use during the day for a drop-in center and in the evening for meetings and support groups.

After months of unsuccessful searching by HERO, members of St. John's United Methodist Church and the Metropolitan Community Church (MCC), two congregations that share a church building, offered their facilities. The center opened at that location on July 16, 1990, with the use of an office/

kitchen, a large social hall, and two smaller rooms for rest and relaxation.

## Organization, Operation, and Resources

The center, which operates weekday afternoons between noon and 5:00 P.M., provides free lunch, snacks, and soft drinks during the day as well as music, coffee and tea, and games in the social hall. The smaller rooms are equipped with a television and comfortable chairs. Volunteers teach weekly sculpting and photography classes; free hair styling is available by appointment. The staff hopes to offer additional programs soon—including aerobics, drama, massage, discussion groups, and others. A bequest left to HERO funds operations, including a salary for a coordinator.

**It's important to check local building ordinances—especially as they relate to zoning, fire, and safety—to ensure that your building meets the regulations. Inform your local fire, police, and health departments about your project. If the day center is located in a residential area, be sure the neighbors understand what you're doing.**

## BRYAN'S HOUSE • Dallas, TX

Open Arms, Inc., offers free community-based, family-centered support services to women, children, and families affected by HIV. Open Arms runs Bryan's House, a non-acute and sub-acute care facility offering day-care, respite care, and residential care to children.

## Background and Development

In June 1987, Chaplain Stefanie Held and Nurse Lydia Allen recognized the need for care for HIV-infected children. They incorporated Open Arms in 1988, recruited community leaders to serve as board members, obtained 501 (C)(3) status from the Internal Revenue Service, and renovated an old two-story home in Dallas close to the hospitals. Bryan's House, named after the first perinatally-acquired pediatric fatality to HIV in the Dallas/Fort Worth area, opened on November 20, 1988.

The Texas Department of Human Services licensed the home as a foster-group facility for twelve children at any given time. Soon, however, the staff realized that the home wasn't large enough to accommodate all who needed its services. On March 1, 1990, Open Arms, Inc., officially began an expansion project and constructed a two-story building on a lot adjacent to the original site. Connected to the old building, this addition brought the total space to 5,600 square feet and increased the resident capacity to thirty-four children.

## Organization, Operations, and Resources

The free child care, respite care, and family support services offered by Bryan's House also include transportation to medical appointments, coun-

*"Here, entire families affected by AIDS receive emotional support as well as diapers, formula, medicine, and even clothes. I am continually amazed at the compassion evidenced by every staff and administrative person at Bryan's House. No wonder the children thrive."*

seling, and parenting support groups. This residential care facility provides an alternative to hospitalization of HIV+ "boarder babies." By providing free day-care for children affected by HIV, Bryan's House enables parents to remain employed, remain off welfare roles, and remain insured.

Volunteers are integral to Bryan's House. They attend an orientation training meeting where they learn about AIDS, house safety and emergency procedures, and issues of confidentiality. Job descriptions help match positions with interests and availability. The job descriptions detail the responsibilities and required time commitment. Each volunteer takes a tuberculosis screening test and, if volunteering in the fall and winter months, a flu shot. Volunteers sign an agreement to maintain client confidentiality, and they agree not to work at Bryan's House when they are sick.

Duties of volunteers include feeding and playing with the children, leading them in games and songs, teaching them numbers and how to read, and comforting infants. Volunteers also help with clerical and receptionist work, conduct house tours, repair and maintain the house, and give presentations about Bryan's House and AIDS education in schools, religious and service organizations, and businesses.

Through the "Adopt-A-Family" program sponsored by Bryan's House, a religious congregation or other group can purchase desired items for an anonymous family affected by HIV to make holiday times easier.

Bryan's House is now developing an early learning program to provide educational opportunities for children eighteen months to school age who are affected by AIDS. This program will be available Monday through Friday, 9:00-11:30 A.M. Bryan's House will provide transportation.

# TWO

# Your Program

Once you've looked through the "menu" of AIDS programs, it's time to assess you own community's needs and resources. This section will help you come to terms with what's involved.

## Considering AIDS Ministry

When establishing an AIDS ministry, begin with an honest appraisal of your strengths and limitations and provide an opportunity for your group to do likewise. Use the nine following directives, most of which were compiled by Earl E. Shelp and Ronald H. Sunderland, in their book *AIDS and the Church:*

- **Be aware that AIDS ministry requires courage.**

  Medical science has determined that the Human Immunodeficiency Virus (HIV), the virus thought to cause AIDS, is not transmitted through casual contact, or even by more intimate contact if proper precautions are taken. Therefore, you do not need courage to work in close proximity with people with HIV or AIDS; rather, you need courage to deal with people who oppose ministering to those affected by the virus. This opposition is often based on fear stemming from misinformation and an intolerance of those considered outside the mainstream. Because of this, you may need to handle resistance and hostility.

- **Consider how comfortable you are with illness and death.**

  Be realistic in assessing your ability to work with people who may have a series of acute and disfiguring illnesses and in evaluating your capacity to deal with anguish, grief, and death. Working with people living with AIDS often brings forth your own fear of illness, loss, and abandonment. Being

Many members of the religious community may be insensitive to AIDS issues, but keep a thick skin. You can redirect some of the animosity and self-righteous indignation people have about AIDS and turn those feelings into compassion.

a part of this process can be taxing, but also rewarding.

• **Evaluate your willingness to minister to those whose living situations or life-styles are unfamiliar or distasteful to you.**

HIV affects people from all walks of life, though a disproportionate number in North America are gay and bisexual men and intravenous drug users. Note that some people may feel initial uneasiness when ministering to people who have been marginalized. Because AIDS ministry may involve entering people's lives, learning about their experiences, growing closer to them, and sharing their pain, people with disparate backgrounds and life experiences have the opportunity to join together.

• **Assess your capacity to separate compassion from your possible inability or unwillingness to condone the behavior by which the person was infected with HIV.**

Some people hesitate to become involved in AIDS ministry because they do not want others to confuse their participation with approval of homosexual relations, heterosexual nonmonogamy, or intravenous drug use. Those who minister have a right to maintain their belief systems even when such beliefs run contrary to those they are assisting. For such individuals, entering into AIDS ministry does not compromise moral integrity. On the contrary, through their actions, these individuals commit themselves to social justice and social equality. Often in AIDS ministry, the parties have a mutual, though usually unspoken, agreement: neither person—the volunteer or the person living with AIDS—will impose his or her value system or life-style on the other. The two parties agree to share compassion and friendship.

• **Measure the degree of your commitment to the task.**

The slow and often negative response to the AIDS crisis by some religious communities has disappointed many people affected by HIV who feel rejected and scorned because of their sexuality, life-style, or medical condition. Because of this, when faith communities reach out to people with AIDS, these communities may encounter skepticism and resistance.

To be successful, AIDS ministry requires the development of relationships based on support and trust. People affected by HIV need to feel that others are committed not only today, when ministering may be relatively easy, but also tomorrow when the disease worsens. AIDS ministry often requires offering assistance at inconvenient times and places. Ministry requires flexibility and consistency as you try to maintain a relationship.

Therefore, when considering AIDS ministry assess motivation and commitment to the task in terms of time, resources, and available energy.

- **Assess you ability to maintain self-control as you assist people in crisis.**

  Since AIDS ministry often involves working with people in difficult situations—sometimes life and death situations—commitment to ministry alone may not always be sufficient. To be effective, you must balance commitment and objectivity, so as to minister without becoming immobilized and ineffectual. You need to guard against letting your feelings overwhelm you. Therefore, you must assess whether you and other potential participants in an AIDS ministry have the necessary spiritual and personal characteristics to maintain this all-important balance.

- **Evaluate your availability and willingness to become educated and trained for this specialized ministry.**

  People who decide to do AIDS ministry must be educated and trained in the general area of AIDS and in the specialized field of ministry to people touched by AIDS. Because AIDS is a complex and changing field, being informed about its medical and social implications increases the chances for successful ministry. (The Resources section and pages 53 to 60 of this section, provide suggestions for educating your congregation.)

- **Be prepared to make a long-term commitment to AIDS ministry.**

  Because AIDS will be with us for some time, local communities need to commit to long-term projects. When an organization does not commit to the "long haul," persons living with AIDS/HIV become dependent on ministry and service, only to have that support suddenly evaporate. Though your ministry may change, scale down, or even end for good or unavoidable reasons, every group should fully discuss and understand the importance of deep and long-lasting commitment.

- **Work toward building a local interfaith coalition.**

  AIDS is found in every segment of your local community and affects every faith community. Therefore, when undertaking an AIDS project, consider building an interfaith coalition wherever possible. Community-based AIDS ministries are strengthened and deepened when diverse faith communities work together as one people of compassion and concern. By coordinating the faith communities and the leaders in your local area that share your commitment to AIDS ministry, you expand available resources and offer the reward of working with people whose faith backgrounds are different from your own. Building an effective local interfaith coalition can, of course, take patience, flexibility, time, and effort because the different theologies, languages, and ethical and social perspectives can make communication and joint action difficult. However, the final reward of working with other compassionate people of faith makes the process worthwhile.

Line up as much financial support as possible before starting. Appoint a board of directors motivated to work for the long term, especially in the area of fund-raising. Also, target individual supporters and pledgers. It's important to factor into your budget money for regularly written communication to your supporters and potential supporters.

# Assessing Your Situation

Before you begin a project with your faith community or interfaith group, do a thorough community needs assessment to ensure that the project you settle on is needed, relevant, helpful, and nonduplicative of an existing program. Also conduct a resources assessment to determine if the project you are considering is feasible.

## Community Needs Assessment

Call or visit your local AIDS service organization(s), hospitals, community service organizations, businesses, private and governmental social service agencies, AIDS activist organizations, religious organizations, grade schools and colleges, and related groups in your area to develop a profile of the kinds of AIDS-related projects currently ongoing.

Talk with service and medical providers, people who are HIV+ and people with AIDS, political and religious leaders, and others involved in local AIDS-related issues and ask them for a determination of which services are totally lacking, inadequate as presently constituted, or in need of supplementation. List all responses.

## Resource Assessment

Sit down with interested members of your faith community or interfaith coalition and brainstorm all the possible resources you can place in the service of your proposed AIDS project. For your brainstorming you will need a chalkboard and chalk or a large newsprint tablet and felt-tipped markers. In addition, ask one person to be a recorder and provide her or him with writing paper and a pen.

At the top of a chalkboard or newsprint page, write "Church/Synagogue Resources." Then invite participants to voice everything that comes to mind in a stream-of-consciousness fashion. Jot down on the chalkboard or newsprint everything that is said whether or not a response seems appropriate at the time. Have the recorder write the responses on a sheet of paper for typing and distribution at a later time. Note that responses could include areas of the building you can use for your project, utilities, appliances, vehicles, money, time available within the building during the week, and so on.

When you have exhausted this first category, brainstorm a second category—"Material Resources." This would include the material resources your group members might bring to the proposed project. Note that possible entries might include private vehicles and homes, time available for volunteering, money, equipment, and so on.

Finally, brainstorm the category "Human Resources." On the chalkboard or on newsprint, list everything that comes to mind in terms of skills, talents, hobbies, time commitments, and so on, which the leaders of the group as well as the members of the participating congregations can commit to a project. Consider the expertise of all your members—builders, lawyers, physicians, dentists, other health-care workers, psychologists, educators, business owners, artists, musicians, cooks, accountants, financial planners, grant writers, plumbers, hairdressers, manicurists, masseurs and masseuses, readers, writers, secretaries, young people, senior citizens, and so on.

When you have completed this three-step assessment process, look over all the entries and eliminate those that seem inappropriate. From this realistic basis, you can now assess any eventual AIDS-related project you may wish to initiate.

## Selecting a Project

Once you have a realistic picture of the AIDS-related needs in your community and the full range of resources you can offer, begin a decision-making process that ensures democratic ownership of the AIDS project your group finally chooses. In selecting a project, try to do the following:

- Focus your efforts and energies on *one* specific project with clear and realistic goals. Remember that a manageable project succeeds. Avoid trying to single-handedly "save the world" because such an unfocused effort dissipates your resources and leads to discouragement, embarrassment, and a sense of failure.

- Achieve group consensus on a manageable project.

One way of achieving group consensus is to allow members of your group to "vote" on a project. At a meeting of involved leaders, give each participant a three-by-five-inch card. Ask the participants to write on their cards three local AIDS needs (for instance, housing, transportation, pastoral support) that they think members of their faith community could effectively manage. Ask each person to pick one need from his or her list of three and write a four-sentence statement on the need. ("I think we should work on this local need of _____ because _____.")

Afterwards, ask the participants, one by one, to read their sentences out loud. Have a recorder list the ideas on the chalkboard or on newsprint. To ensure that everyone understands each proposal, invite the participants to ask questions of one another.

Next, give everyone a second three-by-five-inch card. Ask each person to list her or his top priorities from the chalkboard and write these on this second card. (Ask for three, four, five, or whatever number of priorities you want.)

After each person has listed his or her top priorities, invite the participants

**Clarify the purpose of your program.** Will you be a hospice program or a program focusing on living longer with a higher quality of life? (Note that the latter option means a smaller number of clients living for a longer period of time.) Will you give clients a square meal or concentrate on personal support?

to pass their card to the person next to them. Ask the new card holders to place a check mark beside *two* of the ideas on their neighbor's card. Stress that the new card holder *must* check two items.

Have the participants pass the cards around and check them until their original card comes back to them. When the participants get back their original card, ask them to add up the check marks (votes) for each of the listed projects.

Once the group members have tallied the check marks on their cards, ask the recorder to return to the chalkboard or newsprint list. Have the recorder ask each participant for his or her tallies and write the vote beside each listed item. From this tally, you will get a rank ordering of what your participants are most and least interested in.

• As you consider which of the projects the group will select, be realistic about the resources at hand in your faith community or coalition. Discuss these resources and how they can be used in any of the projects for which the participants showed the most interest.

• Once you have decided on a project, determine the structure it will take. Consider whether you will have a single project administrator/coordinator or a steering committee to implement and coordinate the project.

• Develop a commitment form that asks individuals to list the resources they can give to the project. Encourage leaders and volunteers to include material contributions as well as time commitments and services they can offer. Distribute the forms by sending them directly to members, printing them in newsletters and other related materials, circulating them during functions in your building(s), and making them available throughout the building(s) at other times.

• Fund the project initially with in-house resources. Begin with resources members of your faith community or interfaith coalition have committed to the project. Do not look for start-up funds from governments and/or foundations because the chances of being successful as you begin your project are low. However, note that funding may follow after you have a proven track record of service, competence, and commitment. Be aware that many local interfaith AIDS coalitions have received grants from the government and foundations after the service projects sponsored by the coalition have shown one or two years of successful operation.

• Build up interest or introduce your project by having a public educational forum, worship service, or benefit performance.

# Finding and Keeping Volunteers

Countless volunteers battle AIDS. But *who* are they, and *what* motivates them? The first part of that question is simple to answer. All types of people are AIDS volunteers: business executives and professionals, unskilled laborers, housewives, the unemployed, students, retired people and the young, people with AIDS/HIV and those who are not infected with the virus, those who have lost a loved one and those who have not. All these people have come to a singular conclusion: we are all living with AIDS, and it is in everyone's self-interest to join the battle.

Self-interest is crucial to the success of any volunteer effort. In reality, volunteers not only help others, they also receive great benefits— sometimes tangible, sometimes not.

What motivates volunteers? The answer to that question is quite varied, depending upon the individual and upon her or his needs. For some the gains are tangible: earning credit for a college or grade-school course, fulfilling a court-ordered community service obligation, getting a tax write-off, learning new skills and new ideas, developing something to list on a job resume, exploring a new career field, meeting new people and making new friends, learning more about the community, improving public relations between an organization and the community.

Intangible rewards are plentiful, too: feeling good, having fun, easing loneliness or boredom, feeling a part of something important, feeling a part of a group, relieving a sense of powerlessness in the midst of a crisis, having an opportunity to explore personal creativity, providing structure to life, being given recognition and a sense of responsibility.

## Recruitment

You can use many avenues to recruit volunteers: announce the project at events sponsored by your faith community, advertise the project in all newsletters and other printed material produced by your organization and the faith communities that support it; send notices and press releases to local media and other organizations in your area. Provide the opportunity for HIV+ people as well as people with AIDS to volunteer their skills and services along with other members of the faith communities who support the project. Emphasize that working in AIDS ministry is a two-way street—as individuals give of themselves, they also receive.

When people show interest in the project, ask them to fill out a form listing their interests, skills, and resources. On your form have questions like the following: What do I enjoy doing? What are my hobbies, skills, special or hidden talents? Would I like to work with people or do I prefer to contribute in other ways? How much time can I give? What about once or twice a year, once a month, once a week, every day? After prospective volunteers have

*"As a retired person, I volunteer because I need something like this to keep me out of mischief. I have to say, I don't understand why more people don't have a sense of responsibility to help out."*

**Have some paid staff members—unless your volunteer pool is vast. Volunteers will be more vulnerable to burnout and may feel torn by other work commitments.**

answered these questions, help them match their skills, interests, and time commitments with the volunteer positions you have available.

Be aware that some people who offer to volunteer for AIDS ministry will not be suitable. Leaders of your group need to channel volunteers who have inappropriate needs and behaviors into other avenues of service. If, for example, someone volunteers to work directly with persons with AIDS/HIV, but seems to want to "save" or "smother" them, you may want to steer that volunteer to a job where no direct contact with the clients occurs. For instance, this volunteer could schedule drivers rather than drive persons with AIDS/HIV to appointments.

## Ongoing Support

To help volunteers sustain motivation and stay effective, you must watch for the following problems that volunteers face: (1) *Rust out* results from your underutilizing volunteers. When rust out occurs, they lose interest in the project because they feel bored and unchallenged. (2) *Burn out* occurs when volunteers feel overwhelmed. Perhaps the task is too difficult. Or, you are asking them to do too much, and you are not providing sufficient training, adequate supervision, and evaluative direction. (3) *Dysfunction rescuing* occurs when volunteers inappropriately "try to fix it" for those they are trying to help. Volunteers then become upset when others refuse to accept such aid.

As you monitor and evaluate the progress of your local AIDS ministry, keep these three problems in mind and be sure to give your volunteers the support they need.

Because most volunteers have little training in the field in which they will be volunteering and may have unrealistic expectations in terms of their service, you need to reduce the conditions that may cause problems further down the road. So, you will want to designate a volunteer administrator/coordinator or committee to oversee the operations and to help volunteers realistically assess their abilities and time commitment to the project. Moreover, you must provide adequate training for all volunteers and give them a written job description that clearly states the guidelines of the position in terms of duties, responsibilities, and time commitments.

As you may know, volunteer service constitutes a job position, though unpaid, within your organization. To maximize service, help volunteers feel a part of the organization by giving them a clearly written job description. Keep each job description flexible. For best results, include the five following basic categories: general description of the job; job skill level; task analysis listing specific duties; measurable end results (evaluation); and resources for training and implementation of the volunteer job. (See page 83 in Resources for a sample job description.)

To reduce problems for volunteers, you also want to do the following: provide supervision, give positive and consistent recognition and support, give volunteers the opportunity to air their views and express their thoughts and feelings about the project and their involvement in it, establish standards of performance, and provide opportunities for evaluation of volunteers.

Remember, you must not simply train volunteers once and send them out to do the work of AIDS ministry. They need ongoing support, training, and supervision. A crucial aspect of successful and responsible AIDS ministry is the regular revitalization, evaluation, and support of its volunteers. This is the task of your volunteer administrator/coordinator or committee assigned to oversee the operations.

**Provide job descriptions that give your volunteers clear and understandable guidelines for their service. (See the Sample Job Description in the Resources section.)**

## Educating Your Volunteers

Learning takes place on a number of levels, the chief ones being the affective and the cognitive. *Affect*, which encompasses the realm of feelings, culminates in an emotional understanding of a given concept or idea. *Cognition*, on the other hand, is the process of coming to an intellectual understanding.

Information presented factually can help the members of your ministry understand the complexities of AIDS, but often times they need more to grasp the issues on a deeper, more emotional level. Give members an opportunity to share their fears and apprehensions so that they can confront these fears and open themselves to the new information you are presenting. For best results, *begin* with the affective realm and work to the cognitive. In addition, be aware that learning styles vary between cultural groups. For example, an evening of role playing might be right for a Unitarian Universalist congregation in the suburbs, but might not work in an African American Baptist church.

When considering the undertaking of an AIDS project, acknowledge from the start that this work may call forth volunteers' fear of illness, pain, and death; of people who have been marginalized or dispossessed from the mainstream (gay, lesbian, and bisexual people); of intravenous drug users; of sex workers (prostitutes); of racial and ethnic minorities. To help members of your group work through their discomfort, provide a variety of affective experiences and cognitive presentations as well as short- and long-term support groups. For further information and support, encourage participants to call their local "AIDS Hotline" or to seek out clergy or trained social service providers for counseling on issues related to AIDS.

### Getting Acquainted

To help your volunteers explore their feelings about AIDS *and* supplement

Because the dynamics of AIDS education workshops are so intense, you need two facilitators who will share the responsibilities and commit to long-term involvement. Select one facilitator who is a clergy person or has advanced theological training. Select a second facilitator who has skills in group dynamics or who comes from a counseling background.

the informational (cognitive) component you will provide, use activities such as concentric circles, a panel of speakers, and role play.

## Concentric Circles

The activity called Concentric Circles allows participants to dialogue with one another and express emotions—a necessary step in the process of change. This particular activity exposes the myths and stereotypes commonly associated with AIDS. The activity has two parts—exchanging stories and processing feelings.

*Exchanging Stories*

To begin, have people count off by two or place numbers in ascending order on people's name tags. Form two concentric circles. In the inner circle, place all the number ones in the count (or the odd numbers on name tags). Ask the volunteers to face outward. In the outer circle, place all the number twos in the count (or the even numbers on name tags). Have these volunteers face inward so that they are facing a partner from the inner circle.

Next, give the following directions: "Each of you has a partner. Each person will have two minutes to answer a question I will pose to you. We'll begin with those in the inner circle. After two minutes, I'll announce 'switch,' and you will change to give people in the outer circle a chance to answer that same question. Those doing the listening, please give undivided attention to your partner."

Pose question one by asking, "Even if you know some of what you have heard is not true, what are all the ways you have heard that AIDS is transmitted?" Provide two minutes for the people in the inner circle to talk, and the people in the outer circle to listen. After two minutes, announce "switch!"

When the volunteers in both circles have had a turn to answer question one, ask members of the outer circle to rotate two people to the left so that everyone has a new partner. Repeat the process with the following question: "What are some of the things you have heard from members of the religious community about people with AIDS?" When the participants in both circles have had a chance to answer question two, ask the participants to return to their seats. Then facilitate the second part of the concentric circles activity by processing feelings.

Depending on your participants' needs, you may want to formulate alternative questions.

*Processing Feelings*

The concentric circles activity exposes myths that many volunteers have been taught about AIDS/HIV and people with AIDS/HIV and provides a forum for ventilating and processing feelings. Some of the more reluctant workshop participants will appreciate an opportunity to share without being judged or blamed for their thoughts and feelings. Because this activity can tap into deep emotions, especially for the people with AIDS/HIV in the group, processing the first part of the concentric circle activity is crucial.

Ask participants what are some means of transmission they have heard of. List their responses on the chalkboard or on newsprint. Afterward, discuss with the participants which points are factual; which are possible in certain circumstances; and which are false, emanating out of misinformation and fear. To clearly differentiate fact from fancy, leave factual information on the board or newsprint, and either erase or draw a broad line through misinformation.

Next, ask participants to discuss what they have heard from members of the religious community about people with AIDS. Again, you might wish to write these responses on the chalkboard or on newsprint. Ask participants to discuss which points are true and which are unsubstantiated.

Finally, emphasize that this exercise brought to light some myths and stereotypes surrounding AIDS. Stress that discussing stereotypes is appropriate for this activity but that the participants must not perpetuate false information outside the room. Note that these myths represent misinformation and fear and can be dangerous and hurtful to those against whom they are directed. Explain that negative stereotypes have no place in a community of faith that prides itself on advancing a social justice agenda. Encourage the participants to interrupt negative comments about people with AIDS/HIV when they hear them and to correct misinformation.

**When training volunteers, emphasize that PWAs are living with—not dying from—AIDS. Because many PWAs are gay men, volunteers must remember to accept, if not affirm, the sexuality of those in need of care. Such an attitude can be especially important for gay tenants whose experiences with religious communities are often negative.**

## A Panel of Speakers

Panels, semistructured activities that allow people to learn about the experiences of others first hand, offer both an affective and a cognitive learning experience. On a typical panel, the panelists give introductory comments reflecting their experiences as HIV+ or people with AIDS. This gives the congregation a chance to formulate questions. Following the introductory period, the speakers open the floor to questions. As panelists present their stories, participants have the opportunity to see the speakers as real people and not merely as abstractions. At its best, nothing more effectively chips away at fears and myths about AIDS than real people presenting their stories.

The composition of the panel can vary depending upon your needs. Panelists can be people from within or from without your group. Many communities have AIDS services organizations, people with AIDS coalitions, or other groups that provide speakers on request. In addition to having HIV+ people and people with AIDS on the panel, other supportive people (without AIDS/HIV) can tell the reasons why the issues are important to them. Their

*"My son died after only two months of having an AIDS-related illness. The loss was devastating to me, but I have grown to the point that I am now also able to give help and support to others. I encourage mothers and fathers whose children have HIV infection to get involved with the work of their sons and daughters."*

very presence on the panel models cooperation between people by demonstrating that AIDS is indeed everyone's issue.

In setting up the panel, you will want to do the following:

- Allow at least two weeks notice prior to the panel.

- Ask at least two people to participate on the panel because this gives your congregation varied points of view and takes pressure off a single individual.

- Allow at least one hour for the presentation because this maximizes participation. Note that one to two hours are optimum.

- Prior to the speaking engagement, introduce and discuss the topic with your group.

- Consider having the speakers lead a discussion in conjunction with a film on the topic of AIDS. Screen the film either on a day prior to the panel or immediately preceding the panel. (See Resources for suggested films.)

- If you think volunteers may be reluctant to ask questions in front of others, have workshop participants write out anonymous questions beforehand. You may also want to ask participants to write their expectations of the speakers.

- Urge participants to ask questions, but be aware that speakers may choose not to answer questions that seem overly personal or that make the speakers uncomfortable.

- Emphasize that the speakers do not represent *all* people infected with HIV or people with AIDS. Stress that the panel members are speaking from their own personal experience, which may differ from others.

- After the presentation do as much follow-up as possible to explore the participants' reactions to the speakers.

- Ask participants to fill out panel evaluation forms anonymously. Note that this gives you a reasonable amount of information to judge the success of the panel and to determine what concerns you still need to address.

### Role Plays

Role playing helps participants express their feelings about real AIDS situations. The role play "A Family Gets AIDS/HIV" (directions for which follow this introduction) provides an opportunity for people to experience, on an emotional level, a family dealing with a member who is infected with HIV or AIDS. Through role play the participants may develop a higher level of empathy.

*Preparation for the Role Play*

Consider the makeup of your group and whether you want to do this exercise in a large group with an audience or in a small group without one. Once you have determined how you will proceed, prepare six cards for the actors who will participate in the role play. On each card, write one of the following character descriptions:

1. The Person with AIDS/HIV

You are visiting your family for the holiday. You have received a diagnosis of HIV+ or AIDS, and you come home to tell your family members because you feel they have a right to this information and because you want their support. Your roommate/partner consents to come with you to help you through this difficult disclosure.

2. The Roommate

You discussed your partner's intention to tell his/her family that he/she is HIV+ or has AIDS, and you are willing to be present. Your role is to be as supportive as possible, and you may demonstrate your support in any way you wish.

3. The Mother

You love your child very much, but you are very upset by the news that he/she is HIV+ or has AIDS. You tried to make a good home for your family and you can't understand how this could have happened. You feel guilty and hurt, and you may demonstrate this in any way you wish.

4. The Father

You have always been the authority around your home. When you find out that your child is HIV+ or has AIDS, you become extremely angry. You simply can't believe that any child of yours could be infected with the virus. You may demonstrate your feelings in any way you wish.

5. The Grandmother or Grandfather

You have always been a very religious person, and you believe that AIDS is a punishment from God. You fear that your grandchild is a sinner and will eventually end up in hell. Nevertheless, you love your grandchild and try to understand. You may demonstrate your feelings in any way you wish.

6. The Sister or Brother

Though you are rather confused over the disclosure of the AIDS/HIV diagnosis, you love and support your sibling. You try to get your parents to understand and support your sibling. You may demonstrate your support and feelings in any way you wish.

**Explain in detail every phase of a proposed workshop to the clergy and officers at whose church you're seeking to host an event. Let them review the material you want to present.**

If your actors are inexperienced with role playing, you may want to provide them with a structured exchange to help them get started. If so, duplicate a handout for each actor on which you present the following opening dialogue:

*Grandparent (to grandchild):* It's so good to have you home for the holidays. And it's nice to finally meet your roommate. Now that you're home, I'd like to know what you're planning to do since you've graduated from college.

*The Person with AIDS/HIV:* I'm either going to go to graduate school, or I'll be working downtown. I really haven't decided yet.

*Mother:* Yes, dear, I was wondering the same thing. I've tried to call you recently, but you haven't been home. And you haven't called us in weeks. I just wish you'd tell me more about your life and what you're planning on doing.

*The Person with AIDS/HIV:* All right, I think you have a right to know. I have something to tell you. Before I start, I want to say that I love all of you very much. But there's been something on my mind that I need to share with you. [Then the speaker explains by using Option A or Option B.] *Option A:* Over the last few weeks I've been feeling pretty tired, so I decided to have a physical examination. The doctor thought it advisable to have a blood test taken. I got the results back a few days ago, and I tested positive for HIV, the virus that causes AIDS. *Option B:* Two years ago I was feeling pretty tired, so I decided to have a physical examination. The doctor thought it advisable to have a blood test taken. Soon afterwards I got the results back, and I tested positive for HIV, the virus that causes AIDS. I didn't tell you then because I still felt pretty good and I didn't want to worry you. Two weeks ago, however, I went to the hospital with pneumocystis pneumonia and was diagnosed with full-blown AIDS.

*Presentation of the Role Play*

At the beginning of the role-play activity, ask for six volunteer actors. Give each actor the appropriate character card. Tell the actors that in this role play the six characters are gathered around a table for a holiday dinner. Then say something like the following: "You each have your roles on your card with general guidelines. Try to become the person described on your card as best you can. When we begin, you play out your part by initiating or by reacting to whatever is said. Remember, become the person on your card."

Give the actors a few minutes to read their cards and to think about how they will act out their roles. If necessary, give them the structured model you duplicated. While the volunteers are preparing, say something like the following to the audience: "As you view this role play, imagine yourself in the roles. Stay in touch with the feelings these roles bring up in you. Try to name the feelings: Are you uncomfortable? energized? relaxed? depressed? outraged? Do you have some other feeling? Also, try to remember back to a time in your life that brought up similar feelings."

When everyone is ready, begin the role play. Continue the role play until you feel comfortable that it has reached a natural termination point or until a prearranged time limit has been reached.

*Processing of the Role Play*

After the role play ask the audience questions like the following: "What were you feeling as you watched this?" "What did you feel toward the characters—the person with AIDS/HIV, the roommate, the mother, the father, the grandparent, the sibling?" "What made you feel this way?" "Did the role play bring up another time in your own life when you had similar feelings?" "With which of the actors did you most identify and why?"

Next, ask the actors, one by one, how they felt in their roles. Use questions like the following: "What feelings came up for you?" "Did anything happen in the role play or did you find yourself saying something that surprised you?"

Conclude the role-play activity by asking the actors and audience for additional comments.

## Sharing Information

Though AIDS is an extremely complex issue requiring examination from many angles, your initial educational efforts need not be overly detailed or scientific. With a basic knowledge, volunteers can grasp the issues and become motivated to seek additional information on their own. Members of your faith community or interfaith coalition will feel comfortable with basic scientific concepts.

You will want to cover the following points in the cognitive presentation of your project: component structures and functions of the human immune system; what is known about the Human Immunodeficiency Virus (HIV); HIV testing procedures; the definition of AIDS; means of transmission and preventative measures; a list and classification of the "opportunistic infections" common in AIDS; drug therapies used against the virus itself and against the opportunistic infections; therapies used in an attempt to boost the immune system; and the design of clinical trials.

Since the area of AIDS covers much more than medicine, a basic educational component should also include a political and social history of the global ramifications of AIDS—demographics; governmental, societal, and individual responses to AIDS; educational efforts; issues of housing and insurance; incidents of discrimination; access to health care; and a movement toward universal health care.

**Don't assume that everyone knows the basic facts about AIDS. Be aware that myths and misunderstandings still exist. And don't expect big attitudinal changes overnight. Remember that being a part of the solution instead of being a part of the problem is an excellent start.**

**Work hard to establish effective volunteer coordination and donor record systems in the very beginning. Think through all aspects of the project as much as possible and divide up the tasks.**

The Resources section of this manual provides you with information on the above topics. Included in Resources is a list of videos, films, and books; a glossary of terms; a list of AIDS acronyms; and the addresses of organizations that can offer you help.

Your volunteers, might benefit from keeping a journal. Writing down thoughts and feelings often helps people understand their reactions and fears. Suggest that volunteers use their journals in one of the following ways: to keep notes about the educational presentations and their readings on the topic; to express and clarify their feelings about the material; to carry on a written dialogue with the project coordinator giving comments or thoughts concerning the subject matter; or to keep a scrapbook of newspaper or magazine articles, clippings, pictures, and other materials relating to the topic. Note that these journals enable the project coordinator to stay on top of concerns that members of the ministry group, particularly the less vocal members, may have.

# THREE

# The Big Picture

While your local program can do much to enrich the lives of PWAs, you can also get involved on a broader level. The legislation affecting PWAs and their loved ones is constantly changing. Start by reading through this section and familiarizing yourself with the larger issues.

## Understanding Social Justice and AIDS

This section outlines issues and highlights strategies that individuals, faith communities, and interfaith coalitions can consider and use to advance the social-justice agenda related to AIDS. You'll discover here a variety of options, some more controversial than others. Though certain options might seem inappropriate for your group at this time, you may want to utilize them in the future.

Appropriate responses to this social-justice agenda range from helping people with AIDS meet their day-to-day needs, to initiating change by working within existing systems, to confronting the system from without in the hope of influencing policy decisions. Strategies include writing letters to legislators, taking a public policy-maker to lunch, testifying at school-board hearings, picketing at the statehouse, and demonstrating in a nonviolent manner.

During the last decade, AIDS has been a highly controversial disease that has forced us to do the following:

- examine the inherent inequities in the health-care delivery system in this and other countries;

- consider the ethics of medical research as it is presently conducted;

- question traditional relationships between health-care workers and the people they are meant to serve;

- watch people already considered outside the mainstream become further marginalized;

- accept AIDS as a multifaceted issue that crosses geographic boundaries and has both *micro* and *macro* implications.

On the *micro* level, individuals and religious organizations concentrate their energies on matters relating to the local community; on the *macro* level, the faith community considers the global implications of AIDS. For many people, delivering food to a person with AIDS seems somehow easier and less anxiety-producing than getting involved in the political system.

Both strategies, however, are equally valuable and rewarding. Some people can emulate Mother Teresa and spiritually focus their energies and actions on immediate and local human needs; others can imitate Father Berrigan and struggle within the political arena to change the structure and values of society itself.

However you involve yourself with AIDS—on a *micro* or on a *macro* level— the following pages will provide food for thought.

## Getting Involved in the Political Process

*Politics equals power.* In terms of AIDS, power translates into control over the amount of funds allocated and precisely how and where that money is spent. Power also centers around control over important policy decisions that directly and indirectly affect people's lives.

AIDS ministry *supplements* coordinated and compassionate government action, but cannot *replace* such action. But *communities of faith can have a profound impact on officials in setting AIDS public policy*. This holds true whether the officials are from government, business, or the medical sector.

To date, a unified and committed effort has not come from government ranks. Dr. C. Everett Koop, U.S. Surgeon General from 1981 to 1989, reported that he encountered "considerable opposition with the [Federal] administration" in his efforts to promote effective AIDS education. Even the government's own National Commission on AIDS has soundly criticized the lack of leadership coming from both the Reagan and Bush administrations. The Commission found that "coordination of the [government's] efforts is the missing link to an effective national strategy" and characterized the national AIDS policy, even into 1991, as "an orchestra without a conductor."

Many officials believe that the only people interested in AIDS are those directly connected to the field of public health; members of the gay, lesbian, and bisexual communities; and people with AIDS/HIV. Many public officials, who have grown accustomed to hearing from members of these groups, brand them as special interest groups in order to dismiss their concerns as "not representing the true wishes of their constituency." On the other hand, many officials find that disregarding progressive voices on AIDS-related issues is more difficult when these voices emanate from organized faith communities. Therefore, your group's voice affirming the morality of standing with persons with AIDS/HIV needs to be heard by those in positions of power and authority.

In actuality, you have more credibility and more potential to wield influence than you might think. Government officials listen when faith communities speak compassionately together and when they join in coalition with other groups—communities of faith, women's groups, labor organizations, coalitions of people with AIDS, multicultural "Rainbow" coalitions, AIDS service organizations, AIDS activist groups, lesbian/gay/bisexual organizations, and others. By multiplying your voice, you increase your influence.

The General Assembly of the Unitarian Universalist Association has repeatedly and publicly gone on record affirming the need for a systematic and compassionate response by society to the AIDS/HIV pandemic. Beginning in 1986 when their delegate body passed a resolution opposing discrimination against persons living with AIDS, the denomination has passed a variety of other public resolutions urging the following: 1) an intensive search for treatments, cures, and prevention; 2) the availability of new and experimental drugs and alternative therapies; 3) noncoercive, voluntary, and anonymous testing; 4) the involvement of religious communities in direct service and care for individuals affected by AIDS/HIV; 5) expanded and explicit education programs that focus on reducing the public's risk and exposure; 6) the right of infected individuals to die with dignity; 7) the right of infected individuals to travel at will and not fear imprisonment, deportation, or rejection by immigration officials; and 8) insurance reform that ensures adequate health coverage for all infected individuals.

As you read through this section, remember that a whole range of AIDS services and organizations appears at the back of Resources, with complete addresses and phone numbers for easy reference.

## Accountability of Elected Officials: The Issue

Those involved in the battle against AIDS are accustomed to hearing, "We simply don't have the money for AIDS"—from the White House to the State House to the Mayor's Office. Yet the 1991 Federal AIDS budget was smaller than money set aside for the space station "Freedom." As Dr. Mervyn F. Silverman, president of the American Foundation for AIDS Research has said, "When we saw a crisis [in the Persian Gulf] we dealt with it, and cost was not the issue. We have a war in the United States right now, but all we hear about is how much it's costing."

Vito Russo, media critic and AIDS activist, put the AIDS budget into perspective when he wrote that "more media attention and federal funding ($22 million) was heaped upon the Tylenol murders in one week than on the AIDS crisis in the first *three* years of its existence." Many believe that the government's response has been slow because a disproportionate number of people with AIDS are members of disenfranchised groups: gay and bisexual men, drug users, people of color, poor people, and sex workers (prostitutes). Randy Shilts—the only reporter in America on a full-time AIDS beat during the 1980s at the *San Francisco Chronicle*—has said in his book *And the Band Played On* that "no one cared because it was homosexuals who were dying. Nobody came out and said it was all right for gays to drop dead; it was just that homosexuals didn't seem to warrant the kind of urgent concern another set of victims would engender . . . . Scientists didn't care because there was little glory, fame, and funding to be had in this field."

What is needed to defeat AIDS is something analogous to the government's commitment to putting "a man on the moon" in the early stages of our space program. We need a coordinated commitment coming from all levels of government and endowed with whatever is necessary to get the job done.

Some maintain that spending for AIDS takes money away from other important medical and social programs. A more appropriate response would be that, in general, we are not spending nearly enough on medical research and health care. Instead of competing for a small piece of a limited pie, people must join together to demand a larger pie.

In truth, money spent on AIDS has already paid dividends and will continue to do so. As we break the AIDS code, we begin to unlock the long-held secrets of the human immune system. This in turn will enable us to understand better the broader area of disease and the workings of the human body. Advancements in AIDS will translate into advancements in biomedicine and genetics and will give new impetus to research in sexual behavior and IV drug dependency.

## Accountability of Elected Officials: Strategies for Action

As you become active in the electoral political system you will want to consider the following actions:

- Work and vote for candidates who propose a proactive and compassionate agenda in the battle against AIDS. Attend candidates' nights in your area. Invite candidates to talk to your faith communities and press them on their positions on important issues including AIDS.

- Keep abreast of bills in the legislature; lobby for passage of progressive and proactive bills related to AIDS. Remember that bills specifically related to AIDS are not the only ones that directly affect people with AIDS. Study carefully those bills dealing with other entitlements like medicare payments, supplementary security income, welfare payments, and appropriations for health care in general. Also consider measures related to insurance, housing, health education, medical research, and drug treatment.

- Lobby elected and appointed officials to sensitize them to the issue of AIDS. Ask them to introduce a piece of legislation or to vote in favor or against a certain bill. Survey officials on their positions. Write letters, develop mailing lists, and organize letter-writing campaigns. Make phone calls and organize "phone banks" or "phone trees" (systems of organizing a large number of people to call officials on particular items of concern). Testify at hearings and meetings. Visit officials, take them to lunch, and invite them to talk to your faith community.

- Follow up by formally thanking elected and appointed officials when they respond compassionately to the issue of AIDS and notify them of your concerns when they act in ways that are contrary to your stated agenda of social justice and social equality. Again, write, call, or make a personal visit.

- To bring the issue to a higher level of public attention, send out press releases or call a press conference to present your views and concerns to the media. Organize a petition drive to place the issue before the voters in the next election. Using creative visual devices (such as posters, banners, costumes), stage a nonviolent protest demonstration at a site associated with an opposing official. Note that this action will publicize the issue at hand and the official's inadequate or unreasonable response to it.

- Contact ANIN and other advocates from faith communities and be in touch with your own faith tradition's representatives in Washington, DC, to keep abreast of what is happening in your denomination or group. Be aware that most faith traditions have experienced public policy advocates who will bring your concerns to public officials.

- If you live in Canada, contact the Canadian AIDS Society (CAS). CAS is an umbrella organization representing some fifty Canadian community-based AIDS-HIV service organizations and agencies from all provinces. Based in Ottawa, CAS acts as a lobbying group that keeps abreast of all Canadian AIDS/HIV issues and would be able to provide you with information and suggested actions.

- Run for an elected office or lobby for an appointed office yourself. Consider your strengths and talents (some of which may be unused or untried) and your high degree of sensitivity to matters that affect people's lives. Remember that you do not need to be formally trained in the law or in government management to be a perfect candidate for public service.

## Mandatory Testing and HIV-Related Discrimination: The Issue

What is the relationship between public health and civil liberties? What powers should social institutions—both public and private—have to establish and enforce mandatory HIV testing policies? And in light of such policies, what potential exists for wide scale infringements of individual liberties, autonomy, and privacy?

AIDS brings these questions, ripe with ethical considerations, to the forefront of public debate. Using the argument that the general public good would be better served, many people demand mandatory screening of select populations: people applying for marriage licenses; hospital patients; military recruits; health-care and child-care workers (including doctors and nurses); food handlers; people applying for medical and life insurance; sexual partners of people known to be infected; members of the gay, lesbian, and bisexual communities; sex workers (prostitutes); known injecting drug users; and so on.

Some argue that health-care workers should have the right to test all patients in line for invasive procedures in which blood might be exposed. But doctors cannot ensure that a person's HIV status will not circulate throughout an entire hospital or medical center; once one person knows, the information is easily transmitted to others. To protect themselves against contracting HIV when dealing with patients, all health-care workers should practice "universal precautions": they should assume every patient they treat is infected with the virus and take adequate protective measures.

Ideally, we need to establish more alternative testing sites in which people are tested voluntarily and anonymously. Along with the test, clients would receive counseling and, if needed, information on treatment for drug dependency and HIV-related treatment options.

Two primary questions remain. The first asks, "Does mandatory testing actually protect the public health?" Many think not. If people received treatment for drug dependency on demand, if no one carrying HIV was feared or discriminated against, if everyone—irrespective of social or economic standing—had access to counseling and to promising drug therapies to delay the onset of disease, if a cure existed for AIDS, then perhaps mandatory testing would protect the public. However, wide scale discrimination against anyone suspected of carrying HIV exists in public accommodations, schools, businesses, the military, and government. Also, many people do not have access to quality medical and psychological health care services. Therefore, compulsory HIV testing policies are not only counterproductive, but also unfair for the following reasons:

- Institutions often use such policies as a smoke screen to mask their general inaction in the area of AIDS.

- Mandatory testing can create an environment of misunderstanding and panic by sending out the message that HIV is more easily communicated than it actually is. In reality, HIV is an *infectious*, not a *contagious*, agent. One is infected in specific ways (intimate unprotected sexual contact, through IV needles, transmission from mother to child in utero). One does not "catch" HIV as one catches the flu or a cold.

- Many think that compulsory HIV testing policies are an infringement of individual liberties and contribute to a discriminatory trend toward people perceived as carrying the virus. Mandatory testing might lead to quarantining.

- Because mandatory testing can create the illusion that people are really being protected, this policy may divert attention from real preventive efforts and actually put people at greater risk.

- Mandatory policies may force people underground by severely inhibiting their willingness to test on their own, which in turn may reduce their life span. People fearful of discovering their HIV status probably do not have the information they need to make informed decisions concerning medical treatments that could delay the onset of disease.

The second question many ask: "What about mandatory reporting of the names of those who test positive for the virus?" The American Psychiatric Association recently summarized the arguments against mandatory reporting in its report "Position Statement Opposing Mandatory Name-Reporting of HIV-Seropositive Individuals" (November 1989): "Although permissive reporting policies, designed to protect third parties, are warranted under some circumstances, *mandatory* name-reporting requirements would breach patient confidentiality without achieving any significant practical benefit to the public health. Mandatory reporting does not assure successful implementation of contact-tracing programs because the tracing of contacts ultimately depends on the cooperation of infected individuals. Moreover, current data indicate that if name-reporting of HIV-seropositive individuals were legally required, many people would be discouraged from seeking HIV testing and would not have the benefit of early access to counseling and treatment."

On our continent and in many other countries, public fear undermines objective medical evidence that shows that the AIDS virus is not transmitted through casual contact.

Arcadia, Florida, is a case in point. In the late summer of 1987 the Ray brothers, Ricky (ten years old), Robert (nine), and Randy (eight)—who tested HIV-positive following blood transfusions for hemophilia—attempted to attend their local grammar school. Despite assurances from medical professionals that the boys posed no threat to the health or safety of others, the DeSoto County school board voted to expel them from school. Clifford and Louise Ray, the boy's parents, won a federal court order allowing the boys back into school. To protest this decision, a parents' group organized a

One way to encourage involvement and discourage resistance in the fight against AIDS is to seek corporate contributions to a program. A nationally recognized company (Microsoft or GM, for example) might donate computer software or a delivery vehicle if asked.

boycott of the school. The pastor at the church the Rays attended notified the family that they were no longer welcome at services. The family received numerous threatening phone calls and bomb threats, ending in a fire (which Sheriff Joe Varnadore of DeSoto County said was deliberately set in several places) that destroyed their home. The Rays then moved to a local motel but were asked to vacate once the owners realized who they were. The family had no other choice but to move from the area.

In another incident, the mayor of Williamson, West Virginia, ordered the public swimming pool emptied, scrubbed, disinfected, and refilled after a person with AIDS swam in the pool and forbade the person from returning to the pool.

Some immigration workers reportedly wore plastic gloves when processing Haitian applicants. In addition, reports surfaced of surgeons and dentists refusing to treat persons with AIDS. These actions forced the American Medical Association to proclaim that physicians have an ethical responsibility to treat people with AIDS.

Health insurance companies have sought ways of limiting liability for AIDS-related treatments, thus increasing the difficulty of many businesses, most particularly gay-owned, from getting health coverage for their employees. Currently, many insurance companies routinely require an HIV test for new policy holders. Also, some companies have been accused and convicted of "red lining." That is, they refuse policies to any unmarried man residing in areas with a large gay population.

Numerous airlines have been sued for refusing to allow people with AIDS to fly. The Minnesota Human Rights Commission, for example, filed charges of discrimination against Northwest Airlines for refusing to bring home from China a person with AIDS who the airline argued would pose a threat of contamination to other passengers.

Results of a Gallup Poll revealed that 60 percent of the public agreed with the following statement: "People with the AIDS virus should be made to carry a card to this effect." Only 24 percent disagreed, with the remainder undecided.

The issue of AIDS-related discrimination and the fear of such discrimination surfaced in the process of compiling this manual. The following quote was taken from a letter we received from a minister in response to our questionnaire. Though we neither requested nor intended to reveal anyone's HIV status, he wrote: "My problem is that I am not in a position to go public about my medical status. I checked with clergy friends, both HIV positive and negative, and they all believe such a public disclosure would end my ministry. Therefore, unless there is a solution to this problem, which is not apparent to me, I feel I need to back out of the project."

In 1990, the Americans with Disabilities Act (ADA) was passed by both houses of the U.S. Congress and signed into law by President Bush. This important piece of legislation, which protects the legal and civil rights of

Americans with various disabilities, includes protection for persons infected with AIDS/HIV. Your U.S. Congressperson or Senator can provide you with the specific provisions and protections of this law.

## Mandatory Testing and HIV-Related Discrimination: Strategies for Action

To prevent mandatory testing and guard against HIV-related discrimination, persons of faith can do the following:

- Lobby government and business officials, and/or initiate petitions for laws or policies that will protect people against mandatory HIV testing, "contact tracing" and quarantine; that will guarantee the right to confidentiality of HIV status; that will ensure freedom of travel and immigration; and that will provide antidiscrimination protections in terms of housing, employment, insurance, public services and accommodations, education, medical treatment, and so on. ("Contact tracing" is when local or state health officials demand that persons infected with AIDS/HIV reveal the names of all those with whom they've had sexual or drug [IV] contact.)

- Invite persons with AIDS/HIV, lawyers, and others who are familiar with HIV-related discrimination to discuss the issue with members of your faith community.

- Ask religious leaders as well as lay people to speak from the pulpit to sensitize people to AIDS-related discrimination and how it hurts people.

- In all antidiscrimination provisions and policies emanating from faith communities include protections for persons with HIV infection and AIDS. Lobby for similar protections in the workplace. Be sure these protections cover race, sex, sexual or affectional orientation, marital status, physical and mental ability, socioeconomic background, ethnic origin, and religion. (For information on policy issues concerning AIDS in the workplace, contact the National Leadership Coalition on AIDS. See Resources for address.)

- Purchase insurance only from companies that have a past history of nondiscrimination against any group of people including gay, lesbian, and bisexual people, and people with AIDS/HIV.

- Refuse mandatory HIV testing of your employees as a condition for insurance coverage.

- Insure with those companies that are willing to reimburse policy holders for experimental AIDS-related treatments once consensus has been reached between client and health-care giver. (Note that a day in the hospital with Pneumocystis Carinii Pneumonia (PCP) still costs more than a year on the drug Aerosolized Pentamidine (AP). Many insurance companies would not cover the cost of AP until it was officially approved by the Food and Drug Administration even though substantial documentation demonstrated AP's effectiveness in preventing the onset of PCP.)

- Lobby corrections officials and other representatives from government to ensure the rights of all incarcerated people, including those with HIV, to quality medical treatment, psychological counseling, and health and sexuality education, including the availability of condoms and dental dams.

## School-Based Sexuality Education: The Issue

In 1991, an estimated 2.5 million teenagers will contract a sexually transmitted disease (STD) and 800,000 will become pregnant. The national Center for Population Options found that "a growing number of teens are infected with HIV and are likely to develop AIDS within the next several years." (The relatively low number of teenagers actually diagnosed with AIDS does not accurately reflect the danger because the virus that causes AIDS can lie dormant for up to eleven years before symptoms develop.) According to the 1988 study "Teens and AIDS: Opportunities for Prevention," released by the Children's Defense Fund, about 80 percent of males and 70 percent of females are sexually experienced by the age of twenty. The report also found that teenagers overwhelmingly reject the idea of sexual abstinence and are skeptical about monogamy. The report urges that schools provide increased AIDS education for teenagers. As a group, this section of our population still perceive themselves to be at low risk of contracting HIV.

The current health crisis has forced everyone concerned with the education of our youth—educators, parents, the clergy, and students themselves—to seriously reevaluate the ways schools teach sexuality education. Among the options in the battle against AIDS is, of course, an emphasis on sexual abstinence and the avoidance of drugs. In addition to this, however, students have the right to a wider range of information in order to make informed decisions. This information can save their lives.

Increasingly, in light of the current health crisis, schools are giving consideration to explicit information and frank discussions about sexuality presented nonjudgmentally beginning at earlier grade levels, to school-based health clinics providing family planning counseling, and to the provision of condoms. These strategies emphasize concerns for health as well as for personal responsibility. More and more local school systems are now requiring AIDS education as an integral part of the standard curriculum. Grants have been made available for the development of curriculum and materials, and educational AIDS videos have been distributed to many schools. (See Resources for recommended videos and books.)

More and more people are favoring such education and advocating the distribution of condoms to save young lives. This excerpt from a *Boston Globe* editorial by Derrick Z. Jackson is one such example:

Who will do for Boston high schoolers what New York City Schools Chancellor Joseph Fernandez has done for high schoolers there? Who here will dare to call for the free distribution of condoms in the city's public high schools to offer teen-age students the only known means of preventing the sexual spread of AIDS? . . .

Fernandez has it right when he argues that teenagers are vulnerable to AIDS infection. Since the infection has an incubation period of up to 11 years, many who pick up the AIDS virus as teenagers do not appear ill until they are young adults . . . .

Boston's public school and health officials need to get their priorities straight on the role of condoms in preventing AIDS, pregnancy and sexually transmitted diseases among teenagers. More than 2,000 people in Massachusetts have already died from AIDS. Who will have the courage to say that Boston's public high schoolers—among the state's most vulnerable teenagers—should be spared that fate by forthrightly making condoms available to them?

## School-Based Sexuality Education: Strategies for Action

To become actively involved in advocating for school-based sexuality education, faith communities can do the following:

- Invite an experienced, trained educator to your parochial school or religious youth group to discuss AIDS and ways of reducing the risk of infection with the young people in your faith community.

- Attend local school-board meetings and hearings and testify for the establishment of school-based health clinics that will provide, among other services, family planning; sexuality counseling; and condoms for the prevention of pregnancy, the transmission of sexually transmitted diseases, and the prevention of the spread of AIDS.

- Vote for school-board members and other local officials who propose a progressive AIDS platform that includes an emphasis on sexuality and drug education and the availability of condoms in the schools.

- Keep in mind that consideration, or even support, for a measure does not necessarily condone a behavior one finds morally problematic. However, you want to declare your commitment to the preservation of human life. While doing this, of course, you want to retain your ability to transmit individual moral convictions to your children, faith community, and others.

## Drug Treatment on Demand and Clean Needle Exchange: The Issue

The population with the greatest increase of AIDS infection in recent years is that of intravenous drug users. While many government officials proclaim their commitment to combatting the problem of drugs on our society, little headway has been made either on the drug problem or on the underlying social and economic causes of drug dependency. Most money allocated to winning the "War on Drugs" goes to law enforcement, rather than to education and treatment. We are losing this war.

More and more people in the field of drug addiction believe that if we are to reduce the incidence of drug dependency and the subsequent spread of AIDS, we must use more of the options we possess, rather than limit ourselves to a few. These options include increased funding for drug education, drug treatment-on-demand, and the establishment and maintenance of a program to offer drug users a clean needle and syringe in trade for a used one.

The option of clean needle exchange is highly controversial, and members of various communities, most notably from faith communities, have opposed it. Opponents claim that if we distribute clean needles, we condone drug addiction; moreover, they add, this is only a stopgap solution. Also, some members of African American faith communities fear that clean needle exchange would result in a form of genocide in their community. Opponents of clean needle exchange stress that we must all work harder to get people into treatment for their drug addiction.

We understand these objections. Opponents of a clean needle program want to solve the problem of drug dependency and eliminate the spread of AIDS. But several conditions make a clean needle program worth considering: Not all people addicted to drugs admit to a problem or desire treatment. For those who do, long waiting lists for entry into treatment programs await them. And even when treatment is available, a significant percentage will eventually fall back into drug dependency.

In 1991, HIV epidemiologists estimated that every four minutes an intravenous drug user was infected with HIV in the United States. Aware of these statistics, people who support clean needle exchange programs want to reduce the incident of infection, which often leads to the infection of sex partners and children. Such programs have proven successful in countries such as Holland and England and have the potential to help reduce the rate of infection in North America. These programs will not cure all the evils of drug dependency. They can, however, along with other options, prevent infection until a person can get treatment.

In an attempt to slow the spread of AIDS, an increasing number of political, religious, and community leaders, as well as AIDS activists, have come out in support of drug treatment on demand *and* clean needle exchange programs. As Jonathan M. Mann, M.D., M.P.H., former Director of the World Health Organization's Global Program on AIDS, said in his letter to Massachusetts State Representative Daniel Valianti:

> During my work as Director of the World Health Organization's Global Program on AIDS, we considered the issue of syringe/needle exchange programs on several occasions. In discussions with the organizers of needle exchange programs and with experts in injecting drug use and human immunodeficiency virus infection, it appears that these programs can be very useful for some purposes. One of the most important outcomes of needle exchange programs has been to establish contact between injecting drug users and the health and social service system. For example, in Amsterdam and in London, needle exchange programs have brought forward a substantial number of drug users who had not had any previous contact with the health system. At that point, the opportunity to provide these drug users with the full range of services, including counseling and drug treatment, is very important.
>
> The evidence I have seen suggests that needle exchange has not thus far been associated with increases in the overall number of injecting drug users in a community nor with an increasing frequency of injection by existing drug users. There is also evidence that needle-sharing practices have been reduced among participants in needle exchange programs and may have contributed to reducing the spread of HIV infection among injecting drug users. At the World Health Organization, following a thorough review of the existing data, an international group of experts concluded that AIDS prevention and control programs should consider the possibility of needle exchange, but only in the context of the health and social services which are needed to promote and support behavior change, including cessation of drug injecting. From this perspective, needle exchange is not considered in isolation, or as a "solution"; rather, depending upon community acceptability, it could be a useful part of a comprehensive approach to prevention of HIV infection among injecting drug users and to prevention and treatment of drug injecting.

Clean needle exchange programs have been particularly controversial in the African American community. While some local African American community leaders are convinced of the wisdom of such intervention, others are deeply concerned that clean needle exchange might encourage IV drug abuse in their communities. Again, Derrick Z. Jackson addressed these concerns in a *Boston Globe* editorial:

> Vernon Shorty and Roy Griffin cannot understand why many African Americans in Boston decry "clean needles" in the fight against AIDS.

**It is a sad reality, but drugs remain a significant factor in the finely balanced lives of many people with AIDS. Organizers are finding the issue of clean needle exchange unavoidable.**

Shorty and Griffin are African-American men of the grass roots. In Dallas, Griffin is outreach director at the DARCO drug treatment center. In New Orleans, Shorty has run the DESIRE Narcotics Rehabilitation Center, Louisiana's largest substance-abuse center, for 20 years.

For decades in Texas and Louisiana, needles have been available over the drugstore counter. Griffin and Shorty said the sharing of needles and the transmission of AIDS from dirty needles is virtually nonexistent there.

"The vast majority of people we interview say they get their needles, use them, throw them away and never share," Griffin said. "They say they wouldn't share them with their mama."

"I have met thousands of addicts," Shorty said. "Not one of them has ever remotely suggested the reason he became an addict was because needles were at the drugstore."

Whether it is coincidence or not, 2 percent of intravenous drug users in Dallas have the AIDS-producing human immunodeficiency virus. In New Orleans, 6 percent have the HIV in their systems.

Needles are not for sale over the counter in Massachusetts. Whether it is coincidence or not, 39 percent of Boston's intravenous drug users have HIV.

No sane person suggests that clean needles are a sole or primary weapon against AIDS. Just the same, no weapon can lie idle against a disease that has no cure nor any universally successful mode of prevention.

The suspicions of local African Americans about needles are rooted in legitimate mistrust of the health-care system. Nationally, people of color account for 42 percent of AIDS cases. They are targeted for only 10 percent of federal AIDS prevention funds.

White supporters of needles are seen as patronizing, pushing the cheapest quick fix for people of color. They are seen as using the issue of needles as the soap to wash their hands of entrenched AIDS warfare among people of color.

Some African Americans call this genocide.

As wide as is this canyon, it can still be crossed . . . . Planning and distribution control of any strategy must go to the community. Any needle program must be tied directly with trying to get the addict into treatment.

Boston African Americans must get past the paranoia of genocide . . . . There is no time left to play ostrich when 80 percent of the women with AIDS and 80 percent of the babies born with AIDS are people of color. At the current International Conference on AIDS, virtually every study showed that needle-exchange programs do not increase drug abuse.

New Orleans, which is 55 percent African American, did not wait for statistics. On this issue, the battle is so joined that Shorty said there is no opposition of needles from ministers.

"If we're talking about genocide, then let's talk about black folks shooting up on drugs with black folks," Shorty said. "I'm as suspicious of white folks as anybody. We have as many IV drug users per capita as New York.

"But we're losing to AIDS and the reality is that each time that person shares a dirty needle, that is genocide. The reality is, if you prevent an addict from having equipment that will keep from infecting someone else, then, isn't the genocide on you?"

## Drug Treatment on Demand and Clean Needle Exchange: Strategies for Action

To become involved in advocating new options to fight the spread of drugs and the consequent spread of AIDS, faith communities can do the following:

- Invite people in the field of drug dependency, including recovering drug addicts, to speak to your faith community.

- Lobby local politicians to allocate increased funds for drug treatment centers where they exist and for the establishment of new centers where needed.

- Lobby local politicians to allocate increased funds for community and school-based drug education campaigns.

- Support clean needle exchange programs where they exist, and lobby public officials to initiate such programs in your community.

- If your state bans over-the-counter sale of clean needles in drugstores, lobby legislators to introduce such legislation and rally others to support it. If clean needle sales are legal in your state, work to defeat any attempt to overturn these protections.

Some inroads are now being made. The National Commission on AIDS, a federally mandated blue-ribbon commission, issued a report favoring clean needle exchange in an overall strategy to curb HIV transmission in injecting drug users. In part, the report stated: "National drug policy must recognize the success of outreach programs which link needle-exchange and bleach-distribution programs with drug treatment."

## Housing for People with AIDS: The Issue

This manual has profiled a number of projects that focus on the housing needs of people with AIDS in various cities around the country. These projects highlight the fact that the progression of HIV disease often makes it difficult, or even impossible, for people to remain in the workplace. This in turn makes these people economically dependent. Their usual day-to-day living expenses are compounded by an additional burden of having to bear the costs of medications, many of which are extremely expensive, and other health-related costs. HIV disease sometimes puts people in the undesirable position of having to choose between buying food, paying for medication, or paying rent.

## Housing for People with AIDS: Strategies for Action

In addition to the varieties of housing strategies outlined in this manual, faith communities can consider the following options to help meet the housing needs of people with AIDS:

- Be aware that in some areas of our continent, the lack of adequate and affordable housing has reached a critical stage. Government has not met the challenge, charitable organizations are often stretched to the limit in their ability to give, and individual contributions do not cover the amounts needed. So, lobby city officials to appropriate abandoned housing for people with AIDS and other disabling conditions. Or, become "squatters" and take over abandoned buildings for the needy, including those with HIV disease.

- Serve as advisors or mediators between the squatters and other residents of the neighborhoods where houses are taken over, if such mediation becomes necessary.

- In a nonthreatening way, enlist the support of the community to lobby for quality and affordable housing for all people in need.

- As members of corporate boards, influence the direction of giving toward AIDS-related charities and organizations.

- Within existing publicly assisted housing projects or in the proposals for future housing, lobby for the "set aside" of a certain number of units for people with AIDS. Note that, in essence, this measure involves no additional cost because the housing is either already established or would have been proposed in any case. Consider lobbying housing authorities on the local, state, and federal levels.

- Request that current elderly housing projects that have vacant units be filled by people with disabilities, including AIDS, even when these tenants, do not meet the age requirements for such projects. (Note that people with AIDS fall under the United States Housing and Urban Development's guidelines of persons with disabilities.)

- If a house or other building has been donated to your faith community, think about establishing an AIDS housing project or give the building to others interested in such a project. Also, consider acting as an intermediary with those who might be interested in donating a building to a worthy cause.

## Government, the Medical Establishment, and the Pharmaceutical Industry: The Issue

AIDS has forever altered the medical and social landscape. It has changed the relationships between health-care providers and the people they are meant to serve. It has called into question the nature of how medical research is carried out. And most of all, it has demystified science by underscoring the fact that people previously unschooled in these disciplines can not only grasp complex concepts, but can also exert great influence in holding governmental and scientific institutions more accountable.

Inspired in large part by the women's health-care empowerment movement beginning in the late 1960s, individuals and groups like ACT UP (AIDS Coalition To Unleash Power) are now pressuring government, the medical establishment, and the pharmaceutical industry to put the needs of people first by committing more energy and resources to defeat AIDS.

Though consensus does not exist on the specifics of an agenda for AIDS based on concerns for social justice, some of the points frequently mentioned by individuals and advocacy groups include the following:

- Creation of a national health-care program providing universal quality health care for every person. (Seventy million people in the United States either have no health insurance or have inadequate coverage. Virtually every other industrialized country, excluding South Africa, provides universal health care for its residents.)

- At least a doubling of the research funds for the National Institutes of Health (NIH).

- Expanded informed consent including the right of all participants in drug trials to review drug protocols (the design of the trial) and to review the results, even preliminary, of the drug trials in which they participated.

- Participation of a person with AIDS on the institutional review board of every AIDS drug trial.

- Treatment for drug addiction on demand.

- Streamlining of the drug trials procedures and relaxation of government bureaucratic red tape.

- An end to placebo trials.

- Speed up of medical research.

- Commitment to and expansion of the "Parallel Track" program worked out by researchers at the NIH and FDA and by AIDS activists for systematizing expanded access to certain new drug therapies. (The "Parallel Track" program makes experimental drugs that are being tested in trials available to persons with AIDS/HIV who do not meet the specific medical conditions set for each trial. This program is an attempt to make experimental drugs available to as wide a group of patients as possible.)

- A rational, comprehensive, and coordinated research effort to systematically target all the serious and fatal complications ("opportunistic infections") of HIV disease.

- A change in the rules of medical trials. (Currently the three trial phases are mired in red tape and are overly exclusionary. In addition, these trials don't address the special needs of participants with terminal disease. Phase I is meant to establish safety and toxicity; Phase II and III are meant to test for dosage and efficacy.)

- Clinical trials must be more accessible to diverse populations. (Government and pharmaceutical-company sponsored clinical drug trials have routinely excluded women as a group. This holds true in trials related to AIDS. The reason frequently given by trial designers is the concern for a potential fetus of women of childbearing age. Women must be allowed to enter into more drug trials at Phase I since one-third of the HIV-infected population worldwide is female.)

- Scientists must design trials that will determine optimal treatments for diseases instead of simply whether a drug is acceptable.

- The Centers for Disease Control must change its AIDS-defining conditions to include infections specific to women. This would more accurately determine the extent of AIDS, assist in diagnosis and treatment, and help women receive the economic subsidies to which they are entitled. (Women with AIDS generally die faster than white men. On average, a white man infected through unprotected sexual activity survives thirty-nine months after being diagnosed with AIDS. Women, on the other hand, live an average of only sixteen and a quarter months after diagnosis. As defined by the Centers for Disease Control in Atlanta (the CDC) the limited and inadequate definition of AIDS, which at the present time does not include infections specific to women, exacerbates the discrepancy between women's and white men's death rates. Many women, therefore, are diagnosed at later stages in the progression of HIV and therefore have reduced access to life-extending therapies.)

- Pharmaceutical companies should be held accountable for their pricing of AIDS/HIV drugs. Drugs must be fairly priced, and both government and the private sector should ask the manufacturers to justify any pricing policies that make life-saving and prolonging drugs difficult to obtain by people with AIDS/HIV.

- Pharmaceutical companies must end their practice of price gauging. They must price drugs fairly. Moreover, people must have access to company financial records to justify the prices they charge.

- Pharmaceutical companies should be encouraged to establish cooperative relationships in the sharing of knowledge, personnel, and resources to come up with better drug treatments.

## Government, the Medical Establishment, and the Pharmaceutical Industry: Strategies for Action

Your faith community may want to consider the following actions as you consider AIDS and the medical establishment, pharmaceutical industry, and government:

- Contact the local office of your congressperson and ask for information about the federal response to AIDS.

- Contact your state and county representatives and ask for information about their response to AIDS.

- Subscribe to journals and other publications that focus on treatment issues for AIDS and have these publications available for members of your faith community.

- Attend scientific and medical meetings in your community and present your point of view.

- Organize a youth science club or an adult study group.

- Consider attending a meeting of an AIDS activist group, like ACT UP, to learn about AIDS-related issues and strategies for change.

## A Final Word

However you decide to address the wider issue of social justice—by trying to ensure that elected officials will be more accountable, by taking a stand against mandatory testing and AIDS-related discrimination, by insisting on school-based sexuality education, by advocating drug treatment on demand and a clean needle exchange, by helping to ease the housing burden, or by focusing on the medical and pharmaceutical industry—one of the first steps your faith community or interfaith coalition can take when considering AIDS ministry is to join the AIDS National Interfaith Network (ANIN). In Canada, join the Canadian AIDS Society (CAS). This organization represents hundreds of community-based AIDS ministries; offers an array of services to assist, support, and guide its members at every step of AIDS ministry; and provides a national lobbying voice in Washington on issues of concern to local AIDS ministries. (See Resources for the addresses of both ANIN and CAS.)

# FOUR

# Resources

## AIDS Ministry Support Networks

### Adopt-an-Agency Program

If your faith community would like to join together with other faith communities to form an interfaith coalition on AIDS, you might want to base the work of your organization on the model established by the Interreligious Coalition on AIDS (ICOA) in San Francisco. ICOA links faith communities interested in becoming involved in AIDS-related work with AIDS service agencies. To do this, ICOA matches the interests of the faith communities with the needs of the other agencies.

Called "Adopt-an-Agency," the program came about as a response to a task force report prompted by the city government. In 1989, the Mayor's HIV Task Force recommended that the religious community in San Francisco find ways to respond to AIDS. The report asked for the commitment of every synagogue and church in San Francisco to adopt and support one of the city's 250 community-based AIDS agencies.

In response, Rabbi Robert Kirschner of the Mayor's HIV Task Force, Bob Munk of the AIDS Service Providers Association of the Bay Area (ASPA), and Bob Nelson of the Interreligious Coalition on AIDS called a meeting of the religious community and Mayor Art Agnos. More than 150 clergy attended, representing Protestant, Catholic, Jewish, Buddhist, and other faith communities. A program was announced in which a faith community could contact ASPA for referrals and be paired to a suitable AIDS service agency, which would match the interests, sensitivities, and talents of the faith community. ICOA followed this meeting with mailings and bulletin announcements at suitable times of the year (World AIDS Day, AIDS Awareness Month, volunteer recruitment days, and others).

ICOA in San Francisco includes over 250 faith communities, agencies, and individuals who are involved with implementing AIDS service programs. The most popular seems to be working with Project Open Hand in delivering meals to homebound people with AIDS. Volunteers staff the Adopt an Agency program.

Through monthly news announcements, and frequent networking events, the ICOA provides numerous opportunities for faith communities and community organizations to interact and share resources.

If you want to find out more about ICOA and its Adopt an Agency program, see the ICOA listing at the back of this Resources section.

## AIDS National Interfaith Network

As you consider how your faith community can respond to AIDS, you may feel the need to contact other groups doing AIDS ministry around the country. The AIDS National Interfaith Network (ANIN) can assist you to do this. According to its mission statement, ANIN is a coalition of religious organizations and individuals organized to do the following:

- Link people of faith who wish to provide support to persons affected by AIDS/HIV by developing and sustaining local, regional and national networks and by collecting and disseminating information and resources;

- Mobilize religious leadership locally, regionally, and nationally by coordinating and expanding its advocacy role for responsible social policy; working to insure the necessary allocation of resources in response to AIDS; and offering guidance and assistance in the form of training, materials, and resource consultation;

- Promote quality lay and professional pastoral care by influencing training programs and offering support, information, and consultation to care givers;

- Advocate and enable culturally appropriate AIDS/HIV infection-related prevention education on the broadest possible basis;

- Promote readily available AIDS/HIV-related prevention education to all people, especially children and their families, in the context of sexuality-related education that teaches the fundamental goodness of sexuality; supports responsible, caring, intimate relationships; and respects the integrity of such relationships;

- Promote readily available AIDS/HIV-related prevention education to all people, especially children and their families, in the context of comprehensive drug education programs;

- Promote the provision of adequate services in the context of drug use, addictive behavior, and AIDS and provide education, care, and empowerment for people living with AIDS/HIV, drug use, and addictive behavior.

- Advocate by direct advocacy and the empowering of others a progressive public policy agenda from the federal government.

To join ANIN as an affiliate or associate member, contact the AIDS National Interfaith Network. In Canada, consider contacting the Canadian AIDS Society. See addresses at the back of this Resources section.

# Volunteer Orientation Materials

## Sample Job Description

*As stated in "Finding and Keeping Volunteers" in Section 2 of this manual, you need to provide your volunteers with a job description. The following sample for a residential program may help you design an appropriate job description.*

Title of Vacant Job

Date:     January 1, 1992
Agency:   Helping People with AIDS (HPWA)
Address:  4400 Maple Street
          Suite 40A
          St. Louis, Missouri 63102
Contact:  Ms. Laura Nelson
          Volunteer Coordinator

*Agency Description, Population, or Services Offered:*

HPWA is a residential program for thirty-two homeless people who have been diagnosed with AIDS or ARC, who have a drug and/or substance abuse history and who, therefore, do not qualify for other housing programs. We provide our clients with subsidized housing, case management, and financial advice. We also run an adult day care/recreation program for clients with mild to moderate mental disabilities.

*Description of Volunteer Responsibilities:*

We need volunteers to design Saturday outings.

We need volunteers for the therapeutic swim program at the recreation center. Volunteers will join the clients in the pool, be a support for staff, set limits and boundaries with staff, and guide with clients during the therapy.

We need volunteers for art projects and recreational activities during the week. These volunteers will assist the staff and offer their own ideas and creativity.

We need volunteers to assist clients in designing and making quilt blocks to honor residents who have recently died.

We need volunteers to accompany clients to the theater, opera, and other ballet performances during the week or weekends.

*Special Requirements/Prerequisites/Training:*

We would like volunteers to have experience with dysfunctional families and with drug and/or substance abuse. We prefer those who have expertise and special skills that will help enhance our art programs and recreational activities.

We will provide volunteers with an in-house training geared toward the needs of PWAs.

## Acronyms

*As your faith community and its volunteers work with AIDS, you will encounter many acronyms. The following list will help you make your way through the alphabet soup.*

| | |
|---|---|
| **AAHP** | AIDS Alternative Healing Project |
| **ABLC** | Amphotericin B Lipid Complex (lapisome encapsulated antifungal treatment) |
| **ACDDC** | AIDS Clinical Drug Development Committee (academic and governmental committee that evaluates drugs) |
| **ACTG** | AIDS Clinical Trials Group (conducts NIAID AIDS trials) |
| **ACTU** | AIDS Clinical Trials Unit (individual ACTG site) |
| **ACT UP** | AIDS Coalition to Unleash Power (worldwide grassroots direct action groups) |
| **ADAP** | AIDS Drugs Assistance Program (approved drug reimbursement) |
| **AFB** | Acid Fast Bacillust (retain red dye but not surrounding tissue) |
| **AIDS** | Acquired Immune Deficiency Syndrome |
| **AME** | Amphotericin Methyl Esther (possible antifungal) |
| **AmFAR** | American Foundation for AIDS Research (distributes research grants) |
| **ANIN** | AIDS National Interfaith Network (coordinates response from |

| | |
|---|---|
| | faith communities) |
| AP | Aerosolized Pentamidine (PCP prophylaxis) |
| API | Asian/Pacific Islanders |
| ARA-A | Vidarabine or Adenine Arabinoside (HSV and VZV treatment) |
| ARA-C | Cytarabine or Cytosine Arabinoside (CNS lymphoma prophylaxis) |
| ARAC | AIDS Research Advisory Committee |
| ARC | AIDS-Related Complex |
| ASO | AIDS Service Organization (generic term for community organizations designed to assist people with HIV/AIDS) |
| ATIN | AIDS Targeted Information Newsletter |
| AVEG | AIDS Vaccine Evaluation Group (subcommittee of ACTG) |
| AzdU | Azidouridine (antiviral nucleoside analogue) |
| AZT | Azidothymidine or Zidovudine (antiviral nucleoside analogue) |
| BETA | Bulletin of Experimental Treatments for AIDS |
| CAIN | Computerized AIDS Information Network |
| CASG | Collaborative Antiviral Study Group |
| CAT | Computer-Actuated Telemetry (a cross view of an anatomical part being investigated) |
| CBC | Complete Blood Count |
| CBCT | Community Based Clinical Trials (AmFAR funded) |
| CBO | Community Based Organization |
| CD4 | naturally occurring protein receptors that enable HIV to enter white blood cells |
| CDC | Centers for Disease Control (Atlanta) |
| CFU | Colony Forming Units |
| CM | Cryptococcal Meningitis (fungal infection) |
| CMJ | Citizens for Medical Justice |
| CMV | Cytomegalovirus (virus that can cause organ disorders, including blindness known as CMV retinitis) |
| CMV-IG | Cytomegalovirus-Specific Hyperimmune Globulin |
| CNS | Central Nervous System (brain and spinal cord) |
| CPCRA | Community Programs for Clinical Research on AIDS (NIH Funded) |
| CPK | Creatine Phosphokinase (enzyme found in the muscles and brain; excreted in urine; measures kidney function) |
| CRI | Community Research Initiative (community-based drug trials) |
| CSF | Cerebrospinal Fluid |
| CSP | Cooperative Studies Project |
| DAIDS | Division of AIDS at NIAID |
| DAIR | Documentation of AIDS Issues and Research Foundation, Inc. |
| DAITA | Directory of Antiviral Immunomodulatory Therapies for AIDS |
| DDC | Dideoxycytidine (antiviral nucleoside analogue) |
| DDI | Dideoxyinosine (trade name Videx, antiviral nucleoside analogue) |
| DFMO | Eflornithine (anti-PCP and anticryptosporidium drug) |

| | |
|---|---|
| DHEA | Dehydroepiandrosterone, Dehydroisoandrosterone (antiviral) |
| DHHS | Department of Health and Human Services |
| DHFR | Dihydrofolate Reductase |
| DHPG | Ganciclovir, Cytovene (anti-CMV drug) |
| DNA | Deoxyribonucleic Acid (protein, organizes cells genetic code) |
| DNCB | Dinitrochlorobenzene |
| DNJ | Deoxynojirimycin (antiviral) |
| DTC | Diethyldithiocarbamate, Imuthiol (immunomodulator/antiviral) |
| Dx | Diagnosed or diagnosis |
| EBV | Epstein-Barr Virus (also called Hairy Leukoplakia and Lymphoma; Herpes-like virus that causes mononucleosis and lymphoma) |
| ECG | Electrocardiogram (test for tracing heart rate) |
| EEG | Electroencephalogram (test for tracing brain waves) |
| ELISA | Enzyme-Linked Immunosorbent Assay (initial HIV test for antibodies) |
| EPO | Erythropoietin (antianemia treatment; stimulates red cell production) |
| ESR | Erythrocyte Sedimentation Rate, "Sed Rate" (nonspecific test to detect certain diseases) |
| FDA | Food and Drug Administration (federal drug-approval agency) |
| FIAC | Anti-CMV, Herpes, and Hepatitis B drug; nucleoside analogue; no effect on HIV |
| FLT | Fluorodeoxythymidine (antiviral, non-nucleoside analogue) |
| GAO | General Accounting Office |
| G-CSF | Granulate Colony Stimulating Factor (immune modulator; raises certain white blood cell count) |
| GI | Gastrointestinal Tract |
| GM-CSF | Granulocyte-Macrophage Colony Stimulating Factor (immune modulator; raises certain white blood cell count) |
| GMHC | Gay Men's Health Crisis (New York), first AIDS Service Organization, 1982 |
| GP | Glycoprotein (structure made up of carbohydrate plus protein) |
| HABC | Healing Alternative Buyers Club |
| HCFA | Health Care Financing Administration |
| HEPT | Hydroxyethoxy Methyl Phenylthiothymine (potential antiviral) |
| HIV | Human Immunodeficiency Virus |
| HLA | Human Leukocyte Antigens (markers on cells, which identify themselves as part of the body) |
| HMO | Health Maintenance Organization (type of health insurance) |
| HPMPC | S-1-3-Hyroxy-2-Phosphonyl Methoxyproply Cystosine (anti-CMV drug) |
| HPV | Human Papilloma Virus (causes warts) |
| HRSA | Health Resources Services Administration (agency of the Federal Department of Health and Human Services) |

| | |
|---|---|
| HSV | Herpes Simplex Virus (virus; inflammatory disease of the skin or mucus membrane, especially genital area) |
| HTLV-III | Human T-Cell Lymphotropic Virus, Type 3 (earlier name of HIV) |
| HVZ | Herpes Varicella Zoster (virus; causes painful blisters and shingles) |
| IFA | Indirect Immunofluorescent Antibody Test |
| IND | Investigational New Drug (status of drug based on animal models prior to human trials) |
| IRB | Institutional Review Board (approves and periodically reviews research from drug trials to protect rights of subjects) |
| ITP | Idiopathic thrombocytopenic purpura (body destroys own blood platelets; origin unknown) |
| IV | Intravenous (under the skin) |
| IVDU | Intravenous Drug User (now called "injected drug user") |
| JAMA | Journal of the American Medical Association |
| KS | Kaposi's Sarcoma (tumor of walls of lymph vessels) |
| LAK | Lymphokine Activated Killer cells |
| LAS | Lymphadenopathy Associated Syndrome (chronic swelling of the lymph nodes) |
| LAV | Lymphadenophy Associated Virus (French) |
| LDH | Lacticdehydrogenase (enzyme that helps break down lactic acid in milk and other foods) |
| LFT | Liver Function Test |
| MAC | Mycobacterium Avium Complex (bacteria found in soil) |
| MACS | Multicenter AIDS Cohort Study (NIAID) |
| MAI | Mycobacterium Avium Intracellulare (bacteria found in soil) |
| MCH | Mean Corpuscular Hemoglobin (measure of hemoglobin in content of red corpuscles) |
| MCHC | Mean Corpuscular Hemoglobin Concentration (measure of hemoglobin in average red corpuscles) |
| MCV | Mean Corpuscular Volume (measure of volume of red corpuscles) |
| MEK | Methionine Enkephalin (immune modulator) |
| MHC | Major Histiocompatability Complex (group of genes that control immune response) |
| MOPS | Multiple Opportunistic Infections Prophylaxis Study |
| MRI | Magnetic Resonance Imaging (noninvasive diagnostic technique that can provide information on form and function of internal body organs) |
| MTD | Maximum Tolerated Dose |
| NAC | N-Acelylcysteine (antiviral) |
| NAPWA | National Association of People With AIDS |
| NCI | National Cancer Institute |
| NDA | New Drug Application (application of new drug after phase three of trial and before final approval) |
| NGLTF | National Gay and Lesbian Task Force (Washington, DC) |

| | |
|---|---|
| NGRA | National Gay Rights Advocates |
| NHL | Non-Hodgkins Lymphoma |
| NIAID | National Institute of Allergies and Infectious Diseases (responsible for ACTG trials, part of NIH) |
| NIH | National Institutes of Health |
| NIMH | National Institute of Mental Health |
| NKC | Natural Killer Cells (large granular lymphocytes that attack and destroy tumor cells and infected body cells) |
| NL | Neutral lipids (any group of fats or fat-like substances) |
| ODB | Observational Database |
| ODA | Orphan Drug Act (1983 federal law for licencing of drug for patient populations under 200,000) |
| OI | Opportunistic Infection (yeasts, protozoa, bacteria, or viruses which cause illness in persons with a compromised immune system but which usually do not cause disease in intact immune systems) |
| PBMC | Peripheral Blood Mononuclear Cells |
| PC | Phosphatidylcholine (the "2" in AL 721) |
| PCP | Pneumocystis Carinii Pneumonia (lung infection in persons with compromised immune systems) |
| PCR | Polymerase Chain Reaction (technique that multiplies small bits of DNA to detect HIV lurking in cell) |
| PE | Phosphatidylethanolamine |
| PGL | Persistent Generalized Lymphadenopathy (chronic swelling of lymph nodes in at least two areas of the body for three or more months) |
| PHS | Public Health Service |
| PI | Principal Investigator |
| PI | Project Inform (provides HIV treatment information in San Francisco) |
| PID | Pelvic Inflammatory Disease (infection common to women with HIV) |
| PIN | Provider Information Network |
| PISD | People with Immune System Disorders |
| PLWA | Person Living With AIDS |
| PML | Progressive Multifocal Leukoencephalopathy (viral infection of the nervous system) |
| POC | People of Color |
| PT | Probthrombinetime (blood clotting protein produced in the liver) |
| PTT | Partial Thromboplastin Time (test for blood clotting disorders) |
| PTAAA | People Taking Action Against AIDS |
| PWA | Person With AIDS |
| PWAC | People With AIDS Coalition (Boston) |
| PWARC | Person With AIDS-Related Complex |

| | |
|---|---|
| **RBC** | Red Blood Cell |
| **RIA** | Radioimmunoprecipation Assay (test for the concentration of substances in blood plasma) |
| **RNA** | Ribonucleic Acid (nucleic acid that controls protein synthesis in all living cells; responsible for the transmission of genetic information in retroviruses) |
| **RT** | Reverse Transcriptase (viral enzyme that transcribes RNA into DNA) |
| **SGOT** | Serum Glutamic Oxalacetic Transaminase (enzyme released in blood when muscle tissue is injured or certain organs damaged) |
| **SIDA** | El Sindrome de Immuno-Deficitaire Acquis (Spanish) Syndrome d'Immuno-Deficitaire Acquis (French) |
| **SIV** | Simian Immunodeficiency Virus (monkey retrovirus related to HIV) |
| **SSDI** | Social Security Disability Income |
| **SSI** | Supplemental Security Income |
| **STD** | Sexually Transmitted Disease |
| **TB** | Tuberculosis (bacterial infection of respiratory system) |
| **T&D** | Treatment and Data (subcommittee, ACT UP/NY) |
| **TE** | Toxoplasmic Encephalitis (brain abscesses caused by protozoa) |
| **TFT** | Trifluridine (anti-HVZ drug) |
| **THAF** | The Healing Alternatives Foundation |
| **THF** | Thymus Humoral Factor |
| **TIBO** | Tetrahydroimidazobenzodiazepine (antiviral that may inhibit RT process) |
| **TNS** | Tumor Necrosis Factor (lyphakine produced by macrophages to challenge bacterial endotoxins) |
| **VA** | Veterans Administration (federal agency providing health-care benefits for people who served in the armed forces) |
| **VZV** | Varicella Zoster Virus (virus causing eruptions like chicken pox or a crusting of the skin) |
| **WBC** | White Blood Cell |
| **WHO** | World Health Organization |
| **ZDV** | Zidovudine, AZT (antiviral nucleoside analogue) |

## Glossary

*The following listing provides information on AIDS-related terms and helps explicate the acronyms.*

**Acquired Immune Deficiency Syndrome (AIDS):** A physical condition thought to be caused by a special type of virus, called a retrovirus, which invades and seriously damages the body's immune system leaving it vulnerable to a number of infections and rare cancers. (SIDA: El Sindrome de Immuno-Deficitaire Acquis [Spanish] and Syndrome d'Immuno-Deficitaire Acquis [French])

**AIDS-Related Complex (ARC):** An intermediate stage between initial HIV infection and AIDS marked by symptoms such as swollen lymph glands (lymphadenopathy), fevers, night sweats, diarrhea, persistent fatigue, and chronic cough. The term ARC is being phased out. Researchers and activists are increasingly speaking of "asymptomatic" or "symptomatic" HIV infection.

**Antibody:** A unique protein produced by blood plasma cells that recognize, target, and attempt to kill a specific invading agent such as viruses and bacteria. Antibodies to HIV seem ineffective in killing the virus.

**Antibody-Positive:** A blood test result indicating that a person has been infected with HIV sometime in the past and has developed antibodies to HIV. It does not indicate, however, that a person has AIDS.

**Antigen:** Any foreign substance to the body that triggers an antibody response.

**Asymptomatic:** An indication that a person has contracted an infectious agent without showing any outward symptoms of disease. The person may not be aware of infection but can, through specific behaviors, expose another.

**AZT (Azidothymidine/Retrovir/Zidovudine):** An antiviral drug, developed by the Burroughs-Wellcome Company, which has been used to prolong life for some people with HIV infection. Some of the drawbacks are the high cost of the drug (initially up to $10,000 per year) and possible toxic side effects including nausea and damage to bone marrow.

**B-lymphocytes:** White blood cells that produce antibodies in the lymph nodes. They respond when T4-lymphocyte cells signal the presence of infectious substances in the body.

**Candidiasis:** A frequently-occurring fungal infection in HIV disease caused by the organism *Candida albicans*, a yeast-like fungus. The appearance of thrush or vaginal candidiasis is a common sign that HIV disease is progressing.

**CD4:** A type of white blood cell (also known as T-helper or T4 cell) that helps the body fight off certain infections. HIV invades these cells and weakens or destroys them. CD4 is also a protein embedded in the cell surface of T-helper cells. HIV invades these cells by first attaching to the CD4 receptor.

**Contact tracing:** When persons with AIDS or HIV reveal the names of all those with whom they have had sexual or drug (IV) contact to local or state officials.

**Contagious vs. infectious:** *Contagious*: Infection communicable by casual contact (e.g., common cold, influenza); *Infectious*: Infection communicable by intimate contact. AIDS is infectious, *not* contagious.

**Cryptococcosis:** Cryptococcus neoformans is a yeast-like fungus that can cause infections of the skin, lungs, and meninges. Its most common manifestation in people with AIDS is cryptococcal meningitis (CM).

**Cryptosporidium:** A protozoal opportunistic infection that causes diarrhea.

**Cytomegalovirus (CMV):** A member of the Herpetovindae family, CMV is one of the leading causes of death for people with AIDS. In highly immunosuppressed individuals it can manifest itself as retinitis, colitis, pneumonitis, esophagitis, encephalitis, neuropathy, hepatitis, and adrenalitis. Symptoms can include fever, diarrhea, wasting, and blurry vision leading to blindness.

**Double-blind study:** Drug trial study in which neither the subjects nor the administering doctors know which subjects are receiving the experimental drug and which are receiving either a placebo or other drug therapies.

**ELISA:** The Enzyme-Linked Immunosorbent Assay—a blood test that detects the presence of the HIV antibody.

**Food and Drug Administration (FDA):** The United States federal agency responsible for overseeing drug trials and approval of drug therapies.

**Fungus:** Member of a class of relatively primitive vegetable organisms including mushrooms, yeasts, rusts, molds, and soots.

**Granulocytes:** A cell of the immune system filled with granules of toxic chemicals that enable them to digest microorganisms. Basophils, neutrophils, eosinophils, and mast cells are examples of granulocytes.

**Hemophilia:** A heredity condition in some males whereby a person's blood does not clot. Even a slight bruise can result in prolonged bleeding.

**Histoplasmosis:** Caused by Histoplasma capsulatum, a fungal organism found in the midwestern United States, Central America, South America, and the Caribbean. Disease is caused by inhaling or ingesting spores of the organism from soil contaminated by bird droppings or other organic material. Although the sites of infection are most often the skin and lungs, it can be disseminated, especially to the meninges, heart, and adrenal glands.

**HIV:** The Human Immunodeficiency Virus, a special type of virus called a retrovirus, thought by most researchers to cause ARC and AIDS. Recently discovered variants of the virus are labeled HIV-II and HIV-III. The French name for the virus is LAV (Lymphadenophy Associated Virus).

**HTLV-III:** The Human T-Cell Lymphotropic Virus, Type 3, a former name of the current HIV.

**Immune system:** A system within the body that helps ward off disease-causing organisms such as viruses, bacteria, germs, and other infectious agents. (Also see B-lymphocytes, T4-lymphocytes, and T-8- lymphocytes, Macrophages, and Phagocytes.)

**Immunosuppressed:** A general breakdown of the body's immune system leaving it defenseless against a wide range of sometime lethal, "opportunistic" infections and cancers.

**Incubation, or latency, period:** The dormancy period between infection of the virus and the development of disease symptoms.

**Infection:** Exposure to a pathogenic agent that ordinarily multiplies and causes harmful effects.

**Interferon:** An antiviral chemical secreted by an infected cell that strengthens the defenses of nearby cells not yet attacked.

**Intravenous drug:** A drug injected into the veins by use of a needle.

**Kaposi's Sarcoma (KS):** A cancerous tumor of the capillaries frequently occurring in the skin or mucous membranes of some people with AIDS.

**Latency:** A period when the virus is in the body but rests in an inactive state.

**Lentivirus:** A subgroup of retroviruses to which HIV belongs. These viruses are generally slow in multiplying within their host cells.

**Leukocyte:** A white blood cell.

**Lymphadenopathy:** Chronic swelling of the lymph nodes.

**Lymphocytes:** Small white cells, normally present in the blood and lymphoid tissue, that bear the major responsibility for carrying out the functions of the immune system. These specialized white blood cells recognize and destroy specific antigens. *B-lymphocytes* produce antibodies in the lymph nodes to attack invading foreign organisms.

**Lymphokines:** Powerful substances, produced and released into the blood stream by T-lymphocytes and capable of stimulating other cells in the immune system.

**Macrophages:** Cells of the immune system that approach and devour invading microorganisms. They usually are the first to arrive at the site of infection.

**Microbes:** Minute living organisms, including bacteria, protozoa, and fungi.

**Monoclonal antibodies:** Antibodies produced by a single cell in large quantities for use against a particular antigen.

**Monocyte:** A large white blood cell that acts as a scavenger, capable of destroying invading bacterial or other foreign material.

**Mycobacterium Avium Complex (MAC):** Also called Mycobacterium Avium Intracellulare (MAI): The most common systemic infection in people with AIDS. It is caused by two very closely related bacteria, Mycobacterium Avium and Mycobacterium Intracellulare. MAC begins as an infection of macrophages and gradually spreads throughout the body. Symptoms can include chronic, unexplained fever; night sweats, chills; abdominal pain; diarrhea; wasting; and localized lung disease.

**Natural Killer Cells:** Large granular lymphocytes that attack and destroy other cells, such as tumor cells and those infected with viruses or other microbes.

**Oncogenic:** Anything that may give rise to tumors, especially malignant ones.

**Opportunistic infection:** An illness that would not be serious in a person whose immune system functioned normally, but can cause serious illness or death when the immune system is weakened or damaged.

**Pandemic:** An epidemic of global proportions. HIV infection falls within this category.

**Parasite:** A plant or animal that lives, grows, and feeds on or within another.

**Pathogen:** Any disease-causing microorganism or substance.

**Pneumocystis Carinii Pneumonia (PCP):** An opportunistic infection of the lungs caused by a common protozoal parasite. It is the leading cause of death in persons with AIDS.

**Phagocytes:** White blood cells that destroy invading substances by engulfing them and coating them with enzymes. Monocytes and Macrophages are types of phagocytes.

**Placebo:** Any inert substance—usually in reference to drug trials in which it serves as the control against which a test drug is compared.

**Progressive Multifocal Leukoencephalopathy (PML):** A serious AIDS-related viral infection frequently misdiagnosed as Toxoplasmosis or other central nervous system disorders.

**Prophylaxis:** In terms of drug treatments, a drug used as a prevention against a given illness.

**Protocol:** A detailed plan that states a drug trial's rationale, goal, hypothesis, drugs involved, dosage levels, methods of administration, treatment durations, methods of administration, who may participate, their disease, and its severity.

**Prevalence:** The total number of people with a given disease or asymptomatic infection rate at any given time within a given population. The number is usually expressed as a percentage.

**Retrovirus:** A virus that replicates using the reverse of the usual process. Most viruses have DNA (Deoxyribonucleic Acid) cores and replicate via RNA (Ribonucleic Acid) in the host cell. Retroviruses, such as HIV, replicate by copying their own RNA onto the DNA of the host, using an enzyme called Reverse Transcriptase, which was discovered in the mid-1970s by Dr. Robert Gallo.

**Safer sex:** Sexual practices that reduce the risk of transmitting or contracting HIV and other disease-producing microorganisms.

**Salmonella:** A microorganism that may cause diarrhea with cramps and sometimes fever.

**Seroconversion:** The point at which antibodies to specific antigens are produced by B-lymphocytes and are detectable in the blood. Blood tests rated "Seropositive" indicate the presence of HIV antibodies, whereas "Seronegative" do not. On occasion, a false negative can result since antibodies to the virus may not be released into the blood stream for up to one year after infection.

**Sharps container:** A sealed container with a one-way door for safe disposal of syringes and other sharp medical objects that have been exposed to human blood.

**Shigella:** A microorganism that may cause dysentery.

**Syndrome:** A constellation or number of symptoms occurring together.

**T-lymphocytes, or T-Cells:** White blood cells produced in the thymus gland that coordinate the workings of the immune system. Two types of T-Cells are particularly important:

**T4-Cells (Helper):** After macrophages summon T4-Cells to the site of an invading organism, they lock on to determine its nature and secrete its potent lymphokines, which stimulate the B-lymphocyte production of antibodies.

**T8-Cells (Suppressor):** Cells that shut down the immune system once the invading substance, or antigen, has been wiped out.

**Thrush:** A fungal infection of the mouth, throat, or vagina often associated with ARC and AIDS.

**Toxoplasmic Encephalitis (TE):** A major life-threatening opportunistic infection in people with AIDS, TE is caused by a single-celled parasite, the protozoan Toxoplasma Gondii. Humans can become infected with the parasite mainly by eating the undercooked meat of infected animals and by contact with cat feces. Symptoms include changes in mood or personality; changes in vision—particularly double vision, increased sensitivity to light, or loss of vision; partial paralysis of one side or one half of the body; muscle spasms or twitching; and severe headaches that do not respond to common pain killers.

**Vaccine:** A fluid of a killed or a living infectious agent(s) administered to stimulate immunity by producing an antibody response in order to protect against future infection by that agent.

**Virus:** Submicroorganisms—pathogens that invade and usurp the functions of larger, more complex organisms thus causing disease.

**Western blot:** A blood test for HIV antibodies that is administered to confirm results from the ELISA test.

## AIDS-Related Expressions

*When talking about the issue of AIDS, your volunteers need a common language to communicate information accurately and nonjudgmentally. Below are terms to avoid as well as suggested preferred terminology.*

| AVOID | PREFERRED |
|---|---|
| *AIDS Victim*—This word implies defeat. | *Person With AIDS (PWA)* |
| *AIDS Patient*—People with AIDS are only occasionally patients. This terminology implies passivity, helplessness, and dependence. Use it only when a person with AIDS is receiving medical treatment. | *Person Living With AIDS (PLWA)* |

| AVOID | PREFERRED |
|---|---|
| *Innocent Victim*— People often use this phrase to refer to HIV infected infants and people who received blood transfusions. The phrase implies that some people with AIDS are "guilty perpetrators." | *Person Living With AIDS (PLWA)* |
| *Intravenous Drug Abuse(r)* | *Intravenous Drug Use* |
| *Intravenous Drug Addict*—This represents pejorative and moralizing terminology. From a public health standpoint, many IV drug users do not consider themselves as addicts or drug abusers and may not see themselves as engaging in risky behavior when they use needles. | *Intravenous Drug User (IVDU)*<br>*Injecting Drug User (IDU)* |
| *Risk Group*—This phrase implies that all people in certain groups are at increased risk for HIV infection, which is not true. In addition, this gives people who fall outside these groups a false sense of security. | *Risky Behaviors*—This phrase covers unprotected sexual intercourse, needle sharing, and so on. |
| *General Population*—This terminology sets up an "us" versus "them" situation. People often use this phrase to exclude IV drug users, gays, lesbians, bisexuals, racial and ethnic minorities, and hemophiliacs. In actuality, these groups are as much a part of the "general population" as any other. | |

# For More Information

## Books

*The following books provide background on AIDS. You may want to consider developing an AIDS reference library for your volunteers as you begin your project.*

*AIDS: Cultural Analysis, Cultural Activism* edited by Douglas Crimp. MIT Press, Cambridge, MA, 1988. This anthology examines the meaning of AIDS in a social and political context. Discuss the lives of people with AIDS and HIV infection, their communities, and their loved ones.

*The AIDS Epidemic: Private Rights and the Public Interest* edited by Padraig O'Malley. Beacon Press, Boston, MA, 1988. This book brings together articles by noted people who write about the epidemiology of HIV, the quest for cures and vaccines, public health issues, the testing debate, the spread of AIDS among women and children, the social and legal implications of the epidemic, the strains placed on hospitals and care givers, and the impact of AIDS on literature and culture.

*AIDS: Issues in Religion, Ethics, and Care* by Kathleen A. Cahalan. Park Ridge, IL, 1987. An annotated bibliography.

*AIDS Packet.* Unitarian Universalist Association, Boston, MA, 1988. This packet, which is designed for easy distribution to teachers, ministers, and others, provides important information and accessible resources in twelve separate handouts. Includes a supplement to *AYS, LIFT* and *Parents as Resident Theologians* and provides guidelines on safer sex, information on videos and hotlines, and AIDS stories for children, plus the fifteen-page pamphlet *What Everyone Should Know About AIDS.*

*AIDS Supplement to "About Your Sexuality"* by Ellen Brandenburg. Unitarian Universalist Association, Boston, MA, 1989. Helps young people understand the implications of AIDS in their lives. The guide is available for separate purchase if you already use *About Your Sexuality* and includes the Planned Parenthood pamphlet *Sexually Transmitted Disease: The Facts.* (*About Your Sexuality* is also available through the Unitarian Universalist Association.)

*AIDS: Trading Fears for Facts* by Karen Hein, M.D., and Theresa Foy Digeronimo. Consumers Union, Mount Vernon, NY, 1989. A teenager's guide to AIDS explaining what AIDS is; how one can, and can't, become infected; what is safer sex; the connection between drug use and AIDS; how to get tested for HIV antibodies; and where to go and whom to call for answers to personal questions.

*AIDS Treatment News: Issues 1 Through 75* by John S. James. Celestial Arts, Berkeley, CA, 1989. This book, which consists of the first seventy-five issues of *AIDS Treatment News*, provides information and commentary on experimental and standard AIDS therapies. The author provides information from medical journals and from investigative interviews with scientists, physicians, health-care providers, and from persons with AIDS and ARC.

*The Church and the Homosexual* by John J. McNeill. Beacon Press, Boston, MA, 1988. Father John J. McNeill, a Jesuit for nearly forty years, argues for a new understanding of the spiritual rewards of loving gay and lesbian relationships. The book gives attention to AIDS as well as to Father McNeill's own story as a gay priest.

*The Church with AIDS: Renewal in the Midst of Crisis* edited by Letty M. Russell. Westminster/John Knox Press, Louisville, KY, 1990. Using powerful personal stories of people with AIDS, this book drives the reader beyond pious pity to the challenging justice issues of sexuality, death, and otherness.

*Epidemic of Courage: Facing AIDS in America* by Lon G. Nungesser. St. Martin's Press, NY, 1986. In this early book on AIDS, people with AIDS, their family members, friends, lovers, and care givers tell their stories about their lives.

*Homophobia: How We All Pay the Price* edited by Warren J. Blumenfeld. Beacon Press, Boston, MA, 1992. Collection of essays about the dangers of homophobia.

*Living With AIDS* by Tom O'Connor. Corwin Publishers, San Francisco, CA, 1987. Written by a person with AIDS for others also living with HIV infection, this is a practical and hopeful book that explores the many options for enhancing one's health and improving the quality of life.

*Looking at Gay and Lesbian Life* by Warren J. Blumenfeld and Diane Raymond. Beacon Press, Boston, MA, 1988. A comprehensive yet concise guide on the topic of homosexuality, covering such areas as the role of socialization, the range of human sexual response, scientific theories on the origin of homosexuality, religious and ethical issues, the politics of homosexuality, lesbian/gay/bisexual culture, the roots of homophobia and its relation to other forms of prejudice, and the impact of AIDS.

*Losing Uncle Tim* by Mary Kate Jordan. Albert Whitman and Company, Niles, IL, 1990. For very young readers, this story illustrates Daniel's sad and fearful reaction to his uncle's worsening conditions and Daniel's eventual acceptance of his uncle's death.

*Risky Times: How to Be AIDS-Smart and Stay Healthy, A Guide for Teenagers* by Jeanne Blake. Workman Publishing, NY, 1990. With an introduction by Jerome Groopmen, M.D., this readable, engaging 158-page book written with the help of six high-school students provides clear, scientifically accurate, and powerfully presented information and answers often asked questions.

*Teaching AIDS: A Resource Guide on Acquired Immune Deficiency Syndrome* by Marcia Quackenbush and Pamela Sargent. Network Publications, Santa Cruz, CA, 1988. Flexible, comprehensive guide helps leaders integrate AIDS information into existing curricula. Seven teaching plans explore the medical, social, and legal aspects of AIDS. This guide is appropriate for youth and adult programs. Includes worksheets, trouble-shooting tips for leaders, suggestions for discussing sexuality in a group setting, and resources for updating AIDS information.

*Twice Blessed: On Being Lesbian, Gay, and Jewish* edited by Christie Balka and Andy Rose. Beacon Press, Boston, MA,1990. A collection of writings by and about lesbian and gay Jews who are maintaining ties to Jewish tradition. The book speaks to the possibilities of bringing lesbian and gay experiences to bear on Jewish history, tradition, family, and community life.

*The Welcoming Congregation: Resources for Affirming Gay, Lesbian, and Bisexual Persons* edited by the Rev. Scott W. Alexander. Unitarian Universalist Association, Boston, MA, 1990. This set of guidelines and workshop activities helps faith communities interested in becoming more inclusive and accepting of gay, lesbian, and bisexual persons.

## Films and Videos

*After you assess your faith community's resources and select your project, you will discover what education and training your volunteers need. Survey the following list of films and select those that meet your needs and the needs of your group.*

*AIDS: Changing the Rules.* 30 minutes. Hosts Beverly Johnson, Ruben Blades, and Ron Reagan, son of the former President, present information for a sexually active adult audience. Describes how HIV is transmitted and its effects. Several people with AIDS are interviewed. Includes a demonstration of how to use a condom and information about safer sex. In addition to this 30-minute segment, a 60-minute version, including a 30-minute panel discussion, can also be obtained. A study guide is also available. WETA Educational Activities, P.O. Box 2626, Washington, DC 20013; 1-800-845-3000.

*AIDS: Everything You and Your Family Need to Know About AIDS . . . But Were Afraid to Ask.* 39 minutes. Hosted by former Surgeon General C. Everett Koop, this 1987 HBO special answers many commonly asked questions about AIDS in a nonthreatening way for a general audience. HBO Studio

Productions, 120A East 23rd Street, New York, NY 10010; (212) 512-7800.

*AIDS Wise, No Lies.* 22 minutes. For younger audiences. This video presents a series of ten vignettes about young people from various backgrounds and cultures whose lives are affected by AIDS. A wide range of topics are discussed—including sexual identity, drug use, and fears of HIV antibody testing. A study guide is available. New Day Films, 121 West 27th Street, Suite 902, New York, NY 10001; (212) 645-8210.

*Can AIDS Be Stopped?* 60 minutes. This coproduction of WGBH Boston's NOVA and the BBC's HORIZON combines interviews of leading medical researchers with high quality computer-generated animation depicting HIV and the workings of the human immune system. Coronet Films, 108 Wilmot Road, Dearfield, IL 60015; 1-800-441-NOVA or 1-800-621-2131.

*I Have AIDS: A Teenager's Story.* 30 minutes. This documentary examines the disparate responses of two communities to AIDS by telling the story of Ryan White, a young man with hemophilia who was barred from attending school by local parents and city officials. Children's TV Workshop, School Services Dept., 1 Lincoln Plaza, New York, NY 10023; (212) 595-3456.

*Needle Talk.* 27 minutes, English and Spanish versions. Physicians and educators talk frankly about IV drug use, sex, and AIDS transmission. New York City Department of Health, 311 Broadway, 4th Floor, New York, NY 10007; (212) 285-4626.

*Pink Triangles.* 35 minutes. Focuses on the topic of homophobia (fear and persecution of lesbians and gay men) but it is also about the nature of discrimination and oppression. Examines both historical and contemporary patterns of prejudice in which racial, religious, political, and sexual minorities become victims of scapegoating. Cambridge Documentary Films, Inc., P.O. Box 385, Cambridge, MA 02139; (617) 354-3677.

*Remember My Name.* 60 minutes. The AIDS NAMES Project Quilt, which has toured the United States, becomes the backdrop for individual stories of love and remembrance. Films for the Humanities, P.O. Box 2053, Princeton, NJ 08543; (609) 452-1128.

*SIDA Is AIDS.* 60 minutes. A culturally-sensitive program focusing on the impact of the AIDS pandemic on the Latino/a community. English and Spanish versions. KCET Latino Consortium, 4401 Sunset Boulevard, Los Angeles, CA 90027; (213) 667-9425.

*The Subject Is AIDS* (formerly *Sex, Drugs, and AIDS*). 18 minutes. Moderated by actress Rae Dawn Chong, this film dispels the myths of casual transmission and provides young people with ways to safeguard against AIDS. It answers teenagers' questions about unsafe sexual activity and drug-related activities. The film provides a powerful segment on homophobia and tolerance and a scene in which three high-school girls discuss AIDS, sex, condoms, and substance abuse. A study guide is available. Select Media, 74 Varick Street, Suite 305, New York, NY 10013; (212) 431-8923.

*Suzi's Story.* 45 minutes. A moving and highly personal documentary of Suzi Lovegrove, a person with AIDS from Sydney, Australia, and the impact of her illness on her family and friends. Studio Productions, 120A East 23 Street, New York, NY 10010; (212) 512-7800.

*Teen AIDS In Focus.* 17 minutes. Three young people—two boys and one girl—who have HIV infection talk openly about how it has affected their lives, futures, and relationships. They talk in a way that easily connects with junior and senior high-school age youth of all racial, ethnic, and socioeconomic backgrounds. Two adults with AIDS, who are shown leading a classroom discussion, reinforce the message. Produced by: San Francisco Department of Public Health; distributed by: Current Rutledge, 614 12th Avenue East, Seattle, WA 98102; (206) 324-7530.

*Too Little, Too Late.* 48 minutes. This documentary focuses on families and significant friends of people living with AIDS. Fanlight Productions, 47 Halifax Street, Box A, Boston, MA 02130; (617) 524-0980.

*Who Pays for AIDS?* 60 minutes. This program, produced by the Public Broadcasting Service's FRONTLINE, examines the tremendous economic burdens that AIDS poses for individuals and for the nation's health-care system. PBS Video, 1320 Braddock Place, Alexandria, VA 22314-1698; 1-800-424-7963.

## Services and Organizations

*The following addresses and phone numbers will help you set up your AIDS-related project, especially as you meet with volunteers and clients.*

**AIDS Action Council**
2033 M. Street, NW #802
Washington, DC 20036
(202) 293-2886
FAX: (202) 296-1292

**AIDS National Interfaith Network**
300 I Street, NE, #400
Washington, DC 20002
(202) 546-0807 or 1-800-288-9619
FAX: (202) 546-5103

**American Foundation for AIDS Research (AmFAR)**
1515 Broadway, Suite 3601
New York, NY 10036
(212) 719-0033

**Canadian AIDS Society (CAS)**
30 Metcalfe, 6th Floor
Ottawa, Canada  K1P 5L4
(613) 230-3580

**Federation of Parents and Friends of Lesbians and Gays, Inc.**
P.O. Box 27605
Washington, DC 20038-7605
(202) 638-4200
FAX (202) 638-0243

**Interreligious Coalition on AIDS (ICOA)**
1049 Market Street, #200
San Francisco, CA   94103
(415) 558-7066
FAX: (415) 558-7053

**The NAMES Project**
2362 Market Street
San Francisco, CA 94114
(415) 863-5511

**The National AIDS Information Clearinghouse**
P.O. Box 6003
Rockville, MD 20849-6003
1-800-458-5231

**National Association of People With AIDS (NAPWA)**
1413 K Street, 10th Floor
Washington, DC 20005
(202) 898-0414
FAX: (202) 898-0435

**National Community AIDS Partnership**
1726 M Street, NW Suite 501
Washington, DC  20036
(202) 429-2820
FAX: (202) 429-2814

**National Leadership Coalition on AIDS**
1730 M Street, NW, Suite 905
Washington, DC 20036
(202) 429-0930
FAX: (202) 872-1977

**National Minority AIDS Council**
300 I Street NE, Suite 400
Washington, DC 20002
(202) 544-1076
FAX: (202) 544-0378

**Planned Parenthood Federation of America**
810 7th Avenue
New York, NY 10019
(212) 541-7800


**Hotlines**

AIDS Treatment Hotline
Project Inform
1-800-822-7422

*Provides up-to-date information on treatment for AIDS/HIV.*

National AIDS Hotline
1-800-342-AIDS

National AIDS Hotline
Deaf Access/Hearing Impaired
TTY/TTD
1-800-AIDS-TTY

National AIDS Hotline-Spanish
1-800-344-SIDA

*These three national hotlines are open 24 hours a day, 7 days a week. All calls are free and confidential. The hotline can answer questions and refer you to local support groups, counseling, testing centers, and other hotlines.*

Teens Tap Hotline
1-800-234-TEEN

*A confidential national AIDS hotline for young people. All calls are free.*

*The programs described in The Models section are more completely identified here—first alphabetically by program name, then alphabetically by state. Both lists include page references. Because these programs are constantly changing, expect new addresses and phone numbers in some cases.*

**Adopt-A-Room, p. 39**
Interfaith Assembly on Homelessness and Housing
One Lincoln Plaza, Suite 308
Boston, MA 02111
(617) 330-9649

**AIDS Committee, p. 19**
c/o Congregation B'nai Jeshurun
270 West 89th Street
New York, NY 10024
(212) 787-7600

**The AIDS Lodging House, p. 35**
233 Oxford Street
Portland, ME 04101
Contact: Steve Pinkham, Director
(207) 874-1000

**Brunch Program, p. 22**
c/o University Synagogue
11960 Sunset Boulevard
Los Angeles, CA 90049
Contact: Sharon Wahl, Coordinator
(213) 472-1255

**Bryan's House, p. 43**
c/o Open Arms, Inc.
P.O. Box 191402
Dallas, TX 75219
(214) 559-3946

**Christian Ministerial Alliance, p. 7**
2023 S. Gaines
Little Rock, AR 72204
Contact: Rev. Don Gibson
(501) 982-2830

**Cluster Housing—The Plymouth Model, p. 33**
HIV/AIDS Ministry
c/o Plymouth Congregational Church
United Church of Christ
1217 Sixth at University
Seattle, WA 98101-3199
Contact: Judy E. Pickens, Coordinator
(206) 622-4865

**Community Suppers, p. 20**
c/o First Unitarian Society
724 Park Avenue
Plainfield, New Jersey 07060
Contact: Rev. Margot Campbell-Gross
(908) 756-0750

**DeWolfe House, p. 31**
c/o University Unitarian Church
6556 35th Avenue, NE
Seattle, WA 98115
(206) 525-8400
Contact: Jan Eadie, Chair
UUC AIDS Housing Project
(206) 784-9301

**Episcopal Caring Response to AIDS, Inc., p. 8**
733 Fifteenth Street, NW, Suite 315
Washington, DC 20005
(202) 347-8077

**Food & Friends, p. 25**
P.O. Box 70601
Washington, DC 20024
(202) 488-8278

**Francis House, p. 41**
P.O. Box 15431
Tampa, FL 33684-5431
(813) 237-3066

**God's Love We Deliver, p. 23**
895 Amsterdam Avenue
New York, NY 10025
(212) 865-4900

**HERO Drop-In Center, p. 42**
101 West Read Street, No. 825
Baltimore, MD 21201
Contact: Andrew Barasda, Jr.
(301) 685-1180
FAX: (301) 762-3385

**Lazarus Project, p. 10**
c/o West Hollywood Presbyterian Church
7350 Sunset Boulevard
Hollywood, CA 90046
(213) 874-6646

**The NAMES Project AIDS Memorial Quilt, p. 17**
2362 Market Street
San Francisco, CA 94114
(415) 863-5511

**Open Hand Chicago, p. 29**
4753 N. Broadway, Suite 1200
Chicago, IL 60640
(312) 271-4175

**Pastoral Care Referral Service, p. 14**
c/o Interfaith AIDS Ministry
60 Highland Street
West Newton, MA 02165
(617) 969-8511

**Pastoral Care at the Wellness Center at Packard Manse, p. 41**
583 Plain Street
Stoughton, MA 02072
(617) 344-9634

**Peter Claver Community, p. 37**
c/o Catholic Charities of San Francisco
1340 Golden Gate Avenue
San Francisco, CA 94115
(415) 563-9228

**Project Open Hand, p. 27**
2720 17th Street
San Francisco, CA 94110
Contact: Ruth Brinker
(415) 558-0600
FAX (415) 621-0755

**SAVE, Inc., p. 36**
P. O. Box 45301
Kansas City, MO 64111-9998
(816) 753-2912

**Solidarity, p. 12**
c/o First Unitarian Society
1221 Wendell Avenue
Schenectady, NY  12308
Contact: Rev. Charles Slap
(518) 374-4446

**St. Anthony's Home, p. 39**
P.O. Box 749
Baton Rouge, LA 70821
(504) 923-2277

**Unitarian Universalist Metro Ministry of Atlanta, p. 15**
1911 Cliff Valley Way, NE
Atlanta, GA 30329

**Wingspan Ministry, p. 16**
c/o St. Paul Reformation Lutheran Church
100 North Oxford Street
Saint Paul, MN 55104
(612) 224-3371

**Yom Rishon AIDS Food Drive, p. 26**
Washington Committee
National Jewish AIDS Project
2300 H Street, NW
Washington, DC 20052